T0214646

Lecture Notes in Computer Science 11397

Commenced Publication in 1973
Founding and Former Series Editors:
Gerhard Goos, Juris Hartmanis, and Jan van Leeuwen

More information about this series at http://www.springer.com/series/7412

Guoyan Zheng · Daniel Belavy ·
Yunliang Cai · Shuo Li (Eds.)

Computational Methods and Clinical Applications for Spine Imaging

5th International Workshop and Challenge, CSI 2018
Held in Conjunction with MICCAI 2018
Granada, Spain, September 16, 2018
Revised Selected Papers

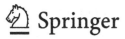 Springer

Editors
Guoyan Zheng
University of Bern
Bern, Switzerland

Daniel Belavy
Deakin University
Burwood, VIC, Australia

Yunliang Cai
Worcester Polytechnic Institute
Worcester, MA, USA

Shuo Li
Western University
London, ON, Canada

ISSN 0302-9743 ISSN 1611-3349 (electronic)
Lecture Notes in Computer Science
ISBN 978-3-030-13735-9 ISBN 978-3-030-13736-6 (eBook)
https://doi.org/10.1007/978-3-030-13736-6

Library of Congress Control Number: 2019933334

LNCS Sublibrary: SL6 – Image Processing, Computer Vision, Pattern Recognition, and Graphics

This Springer imprint is published by the registered company Springer Nature Switzerland AG
The registered company address is: Gewerbestrasse 11, 6330 Cham, Switzerland

Preface

The spine represents both a vital central axis for the musculoskeletal system and a flexible protective shell surrounding the most important neural pathway in the body, the spinal cord. Spine-related diseases or conditions are common and lead to a huge burden of morbidity and cost to society. Spine imaging is an essential tool for assessing spinal pathologies. Giving the increasing volume of imaging examinations and the complexity of their assessment, there is a pressing need for advanced computerized methods that support the physician in diagnosis, therapy planning, and interventional guidance.

The objective of this combined workshop and challenge on spinal imaging was to bring together researchers who share a common interest in spine-focused research and to attract additional researchers to this field. By allowing submissions both of papers on novel methodology and clinical research, and also papers which demonstrate the performance of methods on the provided challenges, the aim is to cover theoretical and very practical aspects of computerized spinal imaging.

We invited spine imaging researchers to share and exchange their experiences and expertise in spinal imaging and method development. Prof. Leo Joskowicz, head of the Computer-Assisted Surgery and Medical Image Processing Laboratory in the School of Computer Science and Engineering of the Hebrew University of Jerusalem gave the keynote speech. His talk was about the recent advances in computer-based diagnosis of sacroiliitis on CT scans. The talk, with full-house audiences, attracted not only all CSI participants but also many other MICCAI attendees on the workshop day.

The increasing number of publications in recent years on spinal imaging, in particular at MICCAI, indicate the high relevance of this topic to the community. After four very successful workshops at MICCAI 2013, 2014, 2015 and 2016, we also had an increased number of participants in this year's workshop. We accepted eight regular papers on spine image analysis, including vertebra detection, spine segmentation, image-based diagnosis, and image-guided spinal surgery. Each submission was rigorously reviewed by two or three Program Committee members on the basis of its technical quality, relevance, significance, and clarity. The best paper award was given to the paper "Automated Grading of Modic Changes Using CNNs — Improving the Performance with Mixup" by Dimitrios Damopoulos et al., based on the raw scores of all review feedbacks.

In addition to regular research presentations, the computational challenge was organized to attract researchers working on general-purpose algorithms to try their methods on spinal data. The MICCAI 2018 Challenge on Automatic IVD Localization and Segmentation from 3D Multi-modality MR (M3) Images was jointly organized with the CSI 2018 workshop. The goal of the challenge was to investigate (semi-) automatic IVD localization and segmentation algorithms and provide a standard evaluation framework with a set of multi-modality MR images acquired with the Dixon protocol. The challenge attract eight participating teams with nine submissions. The Changliu team achieved the best performance on all metrics. The short papers of the IVD challenge participants are included in the workshop proceedings. These short papers focused on presenting the methodologies used for the challenge segmentation task.

We would like to thank the MICCAI workshop organizers for supporting the organization of the CSI workshop, all of the Program Committee members for their great efforts and cooperation in reviewing and selecting the papers. We would also like to thank all of the participants for attending the regular presentation sessions and challenge competition session. Finally, our gratitude goes to Alfred Hofmann, Anna Kramer, and Ingrid Haas of Springer for their continuous support in the publication of the workshop proceedings.

September 2018   Yunliang Cai
Guoyan Zheng
Daniel Belavy
Shuo Li

Organization

General Chairs

Guoyan Zheng   University of Bern, Switzerland
Daniel Belavy   Deakin University, Australia
Yunliang Cai   Worcester Polytechnic Institute, USA
Shuo Li   Western University, Canada

Program Committee

Michel Audette   Old Dominion University, USA
Ulas Bagci   University of Central Florida, USA
Paul A. Bromiley   University of Manchester, UK
Daniel Forsberg   Sectra AB, Linköping University, Sweden
Pheng Ann Heng   Chinese University of Hong Kong, HKSAR China
Songbai Ji   Worcester Polytechnic Institute, USA
Samuel Kadoury   Polytechnique Montréal, Canada
Cristian Lorenz   Philips GmbH Innovative Technologies, Germany
Simon Pezold   University of Basel, Switzerland

Contents

Regular Papers

Spinal Cord Gray Matter-White Matter Segmentation on Magnetic Resonance AMIRA Images with MD-GRU

Antal Horváth[1(⊠)], Charidimos Tsagkas[2], Simon Andermatt[1], Simon Pezold[1], Katrin Parmar[2], and Philippe Cattin[1]

[1] Department of Biomedical Engineering, University of Basel, Allschwil, Switzerland
`antal.horvath@unibas.ch`
[2] Department of Neurology, University Hospital Basel, Basel, Switzerland

Abstract. The small butterfly shaped structure of spinal cord (SC) gray matter (GM) is challenging to image and to delineate from its surrounding white matter (WM). Segmenting GM is up to a point a trade-off between accuracy and precision. We propose a new pipeline for GM-WM magnetic resonance (MR) image acquisition and segmentation. We report superior results as compared to the ones recently reported in the SC GM segmentation challenge and show even better results using the averaged magnetization inversion recovery acquisitions (AMIRA) sequence. Scan-rescan experiments with the AMIRA sequence show high reproducibility in terms of Dice coefficient, Hausdorff distance and relative standard deviation. We use a recurrent neural network (RNN) with multi-dimensional gated recurrent units (MD-GRU) to train segmentation models on the AMIRA dataset of 855 slices. We added a generalized dice loss to the cross entropy loss that MD-GRU uses and were able to improve the results.

Keywords: Segmentation · Spinal cord · Gray matter · White matter · Deep learning · RNN · MD-GRU

1 Introduction

Cervical spinal cord (SC) segmentation in magnetic resonance (MR) images is a viable means for quantitatively assessing the neurodegenerative effects of diseases in the central nervous system. While conventional MR sequences only allowed differentiation of the boundary between SC and cerebrospinal fluid (CSF), more recent sequences can be used to distinguish the SC's inner gray matter (GM) and white matter (WM) compartments. The latter task, however, remains challenging as state-of-the-art MR sequences only achieve an in-slice resolution of around 0.5 mm while maintaining a good signal-to-noise ratio (SNR) and an

---

A. Horváth and C. Tsagkas—These two authors contributed equally.

© Springer Nature Switzerland AG 2019
G. Zheng et al. (Eds.): CSI 2018, LNCS 11397, pp. 3–14, 2019.
https://doi.org/10.1007/978-3-030-13736-6_1

acceptable acquisition time. This resolution is barely enough to visualize the SC's butterfly-shaped GM structure.

The 2016 spinal cord gray matter segmentation (SCGM) challenge [7] reported mean Dice similarity coefficients (DSC) of 0.8 in comparison to a manual consensus ground truth for the best SC GM segmentation approaches at that time. Porisky et al. [6] experimented with 3D convolutional encoder networks but did not improve the challenge's results. Perone et al.'s U-Net approach [5] later managed to push the DSC value to 0.85. More recently, Datta et al. [3] reported mean DSC of 0.88 on images of various MR sequences with a morphological geodesic active contour model.

Still, this means that a high number of subjects would be necessary to get reliable findings from clinical trials. Hence, despite recent developments, there is a need for improvement of the reproducibility of SC GM and WM measurements. An accurate and precise segmentation of the SC's inner structures in MR images under the mentioned limiting trade-off between resolution, SNR, and time therefore remains a challenge, especially when focusing on the GM.

In this work, we present a new robust and fully automatic pipeline for the acquisition and segmentation of GM and WM in MR images of the SC. On the segmentation side, we propose the use of multi-dimensional gated recurrent units (MD-GRU), which already proved fit for a number of medical segmentation tasks [1], to gain accurate and precise SC GM and WM segmentations. To this end, we adapt MD-GRU's original cross-entropy loss by integrating a generalized Dice loss (GDL) [8] and show improved segmentation performance compared to the original. Using the proposed setup, we manage to set a new state of the art on the SCGM challenge data with a mean DSC of 0.9. On the imaging side, we propose to use the AMIRA MR sequence [9] for gaining improved GM-WM and WM-CSF contrast in axial cross-sectional slices of the SC. Using the proposed MD-GRU approach in combination with this new imaging sequence, we manage to gain an even higher accuracy of DSC 0.91 wrt. a manual ground truth, as we demonstrate in experiments on scan-rescan images of healthy subjects, for both SC GM and WM.

The remaining paper is structured as follows: in Sect. 2, we present our segmentation method; in Sect. 3, we briefly describe the AMIRA MR sequence and the two datasets (SCGM challenge, AMIRA images) that we use for the experiments of Sect. 4, before we conclude in Sect. 5.

2 Method

The Multi-Dimensional Gated Recurrent Unit (MD-GRU) [1] is a generalization of a bi-directional recurrent neural network (RNN), which is able to process images. It achieves this task by treating each direction along each of the spatial dimensions independently as a temporal direction. The MD-GRU processes the image using two convolutional GRUs (C-GRUs) for each image dimension, one in forward and one in backward direction, and combines the results of all individual C-GRUs. The gated recurrent unit (GRU), compared to the more popular and established long short-term memory (LSTM), uses a simpler gating structure and combines its state and output. The GRU has been shown to produce comparable results while consuming less memory than its LSTM counterpart when applied to image segmentation and hence allows for larger images to be processed [1].

We directly feed the 2D version of MD-GRU the 8-channel AMIRA images (cf. Sect. 3.1) to train AMIRA segmentation models, but only use the single channel images of the SCGM dataset (cf. Sect. 3.2) for the challenge models. To address the high class imbalance between background, WM and GM, similar to [5] we added a GM Dice loss (DL), but also included DLs for all the other label classes using the generalized Dice loss (GDL) formulation of Sudre et al. [8].

2.1 Dice Loss

A straightforward approximation of a DL for a multi-labelling problem is

$$L_{\mathrm{D}} = -\frac{1}{\sum_{\ell \in \mathcal{L}} \omega_\ell} \sum_{\ell \in \mathcal{L}} \omega_\ell \frac{2 \sum_{x \in X} p_{\ell x} r_{\ell x}}{\sum_{x \in X} p_{\ell x} + r_{\ell x}}, \qquad (1)$$

with the image domain X, labels $\mathcal{L}$, predictions p, raters r, and class weights ω. Sudre et al. [8] described a Generalized Dice Loss (GDL) L_{GD} where they divide the weighted sum of the intersections of all labels by the weighted sum of all predictions and targets of all labels, instead of just linearly combining the individual Dice coefficients:

$$L_{\mathrm{GD}} = -\frac{2 \sum_{\ell \in \mathcal{L}} \omega_\ell \sum_{x \in X} p_{\ell x} r_{\ell x}}{\sum_{\ell \in \mathcal{L}} \omega_\ell \sum_{x \in X} p_{\ell x} + r_{\ell x}}. \qquad (2)$$

As stated in [2], compared to the DL (1), the GDL (2) allows all labels to contribute equally to the overall overlap (denominator in (2)).

The (squared) inverse volume weighting

$$\omega_\ell = \frac{1}{\left(\sum_{x \in X} r_{\ell x}\right)^2}, \qquad (3)$$

as proposed in [2], deals with the class imbalance problem: large regions only contribute very little to L_{D} or L_{GD}, whereas small regions are weighted more and thus are more important in the optimization process.

To avoid division by zero in ω_ℓ for image samples with absence of label ℓ, we regularize the denominator of (3) and formulate the weighting we used:

$$\omega_\ell = \frac{1}{1 + \left(\sum_{x \in X} r_{\ell x}\right)^2}. \qquad (4)$$

The weighting (4) compared to (3) only slightly decreases its value as long as the object of interest has enough pixels. Note, that during training of a network, it is possible, that not all labels occur in a random subsample with random location.

Finally, we combine DL or GDL with the cross entropy loss L_{C} (CEL) with a factor $\lambda \in [0, 1]$:

$$L = \lambda L_{\mathrm{D \ or \ GD}} + (1 - \lambda) L_{\mathrm{C}}.$$

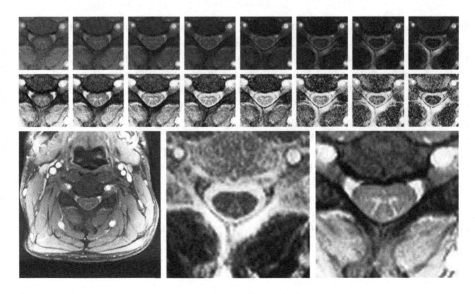

Fig. 1. AMIRA sequence of an exemplary slice on C4 level. All images 10-fold upsampled. *Top and middle row:* Inversion images with increasing inversion times from left to right. Original cropped images (*top*), and histogram equalized (*middle*). *Bottom row:* Histogram equalized sum of the first 5 inversion images in full view (*left*), weighted average with optimal CSF-WM contrast (*middle*), and optimal GM-WM contrast (*right*).

3 Data

In the following subsections, we describe the images used for the experiments: healthy subjects scan-rescan AMIRA dataset (own), which we call the AMIRA dataset, and the SCGM challenge dataset[1] [7], which we refer to as SCGM dataset.

3.1 AMIRA Dataset

The first dataset used in this paper consists of 24 healthy subjects (14 female, 10 male, age 40 ± 11 years). Each subject was scanned 3 times, remaining in the scanner between the first and second scan, and leaving the scanner and being repositioned between the second and third scan. Each scan contains 12 axial cross-sectional slices of the neck acquired with the AMIRA sequence [9] that were manually aligned at acquisition time perpendicular to the SC's centerline with an average slice distance of 4 mm starting from vertebra C3 level in caudal direction.

---

[1] http://cmictig.cs.ucl.ac.uk/niftyweb/program.php?p=CHALLENGE last accessed: September 13, 2018.

Because of severe imaging artifacts some slices had to be discarded. For one scan the last three caudal slices, for two scans the last two slices and for another two scans the last slice, in total 9 out of the 864 slices were discarded.

The AMIRA sequence consists of 8 inversion images of the same anatomical slice captured at different inversion times after 180° MR pulses that have an in-slice resolution of 0.67 mm × 0.67 mm. Exemplary inversion images and different averages of an exemplary slice on vertebra C4 level are shown in Fig. 1. For human raters, to manually segment the AMIRA images, different single channel projections of the 8 channel images are necessary. Weighted averages of the inversion images with e.g. optimal CSF-WM or GM-WM contrast, see Fig. 1, were calculated with an approach that maximizes between-class intensity mean values and minimizes within-class intensity variances [4].

In order to reduce the numerical errors for the calculated measures, we 10-fold upsampled all slices with Lanczos interpolation. Since all images were manually centered at the SC, we consequently trimmed one third of the image size on each side and thus cropped out the inner ninth to a size of 650 × 650 pixels for faster processing.

One experienced rater segmented all 855 images manually for WM and GM and segmented again 60 randomly chosen slices over all subjects, scans and slices, without knowledge of their origin, to enable an intra-rater comparison.

3.2 SCGM Dataset

The SCGM segmentation challenge data [7] consists of 40 training datasets and 40 test datasets acquired at 4 different sites. Both training and test datasets each have 10 samples of each site. The 4 sites have different imaging protocols with different field of view, size and resolution. Each dataset was manually segmented by 4 experts and to assess rater performance, with majority voting (more than 2 positive votes) a consensus segmentation of the 4 raters was calculated.

For training and testing of our MD-GRU models, we resampled all axial slices of all the datasets to the common finest resolution of 0.25 mm × 0.25 mm and center cropped or padded all datasets to a common size of 640 × 640 pixels. Before submitting the testing results for evaluation, we padded and resampled all slices to their original sizes and resolutions.

4 Experiments and Results

In the following subsections, we describe our experiments, the chosen MD-GRU options, and show their results.

4.1 AMIRA Segmentation Model

We split the 24 subjects into 3 groups of 8 subjects each for 3 cross-validations: training on two groups and testing on a third group. To handle over-fitting, of each training set we excluded one subject and used it for validation.

We used the standard MD-GRU[2] model with default settings and residual learning, dropout rate 0.5, and dropconnect on state. We chose the following problem specific parameters: Gaussian high pass filtering with variance 10, batch size 1, and window size 500 × 500 pixels. In each iteration of the training stage, for data augmentation, a subsample of the training data with random deformation field at a random location was selected. Random deformations included an interpolated deformation field on 4 supporting points with randomly generated deformations of standard deviation of 15, random scaling of a factor between $4/5$ and $5/4$, random rotation of $\pm 10°$, and random mirroring along the anatomical median plane. To prevent zero padding of the subsamples, we only allowed random sampling within a safe distance of 45 pixels from the image boundary and truncated the random deformation magnitudes to 45 pixels, which is 3 times the chosen standard deviation.

We trained the networks with Adadelta with a learning rate of 1 for 30'000 iterations, where one iteration approximately took 10 s on an NVIDIA GeForce GTX Titan X. Cross entropy and DSC on the evaluation set already reached their upper bounds after around 20'000 iterations, and dropconnect on state prevented from overfitting as we can see in Fig. 3.

The time for segmenting a slice with the trained network approximately took 7 s.

Prior to the final model generation, we experimented in adding only a GM DL to the CEL with weightings $\lambda = 0, 0.25, 0.5, 0.75, 1$ and figured that 0.5 produced the best results. DL produces values close to -1 whereas CEL tends to have small values close to 0. Moreover, CEL holds the information of all labels, since it is calculated over all labels. Now, when adding only GM DL, because of the imbalance of the loss values, higher values of λ strongly weaken the information for WM and background that in this setup is carried only within CEL. The best weighting λ depends on the cross entropy and thus depends on the class imbalance and label uncertainty of each specific segmentation task.

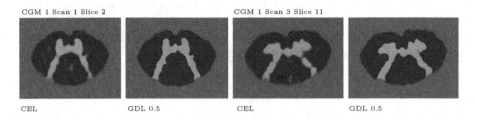

Fig. 2. Exemplary prediction probability maps of the three labeling maps background (*red*), GM (*green*) and WM (*blue*) of MD-GRU with CEL and with GDL in RGB colors. (Color figure online)

---

[2] https://github.com/zubata88/mdgru last accessed: September 13, 2018.

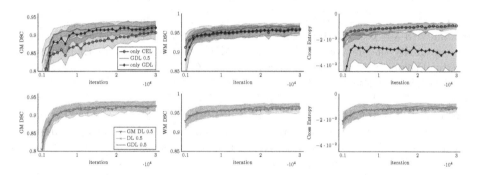

Fig. 3. GM DSC, WM DSC and cross entropy over the training iterations of the validation set of group 1 in the AMIRA dataset in the format mean ± one standard deviation. *Top row:* models with $\lambda = 0$ (only CEL), $\lambda = 1$ (only GDL), and combined with $\lambda = 0.5$ (GDL 0.5). *Bottom row:* GM DL 0.5, DL 0.5, and GDL 0.5 show similar performance.

We observed that the auxiliary DL produces sharper probability maps at the boundaries as compared to only using CEL, see Fig. 2, and that DL helps to delineate weak contrasts e.g. between GM and WM.

Further experiments showed, that the proposed automatic weightings ω_ℓ (4) for the DLs between all label classes is a good strategy to simplify the selection of λ. In our case, the evaluation scores did not show big differences for λ in a range from 0.25 to 0.75, when using the class weights ω_ℓ according to (4) for both DL and GDL. MD-GRU with the trivial linear combinations $\lambda = 0$ (only CEL) and $\lambda = 1$ (only GDL) did not perform as good as true combinations between the two losses. We show the improvement in the scores of GDL with $\lambda = 0.5$ in Fig. 3 and Table 1.

Table 1. Improvement between native MD-GRU with CEL and the proposed MD-GRU with GDL together with the manual segmentation's precision and intra-rater accuracy values. Intra-rater accuracy of the human expert was calculated for the 60 randomly chosen slices.

GM	Accuracy DSC	HD(mm)	Intra-session DSC	HD(mm)	RSD(%)	Inter-session DSC	HD(mm)	RSD(%)
MD-GRU CEL	0.90 ± 0.04	0.68 ± 0.43	0.89 ± 0.03	0.71 ± 0.46	3.22 ± 2.87	0.88 ± 0.04	0.70 ± 0.43	3.65 ± 3.97
MD-GRU GDL 0.5	0.91 ± 0.03	0.56 ± 0.33	0.88 ± 0.03	0.58 ± 0.32	2.93 ± 2.63	0.88 ± 0.03	0.61 ± 0.35	3.86 ± 3.49
Manual			0.86 ± 0.03	0.67 ± 0.24	5.55 ± 4.11	0.85 ± 0.03	0.71 ± 0.27	6.27 ± 4.70
Intra-rater	0.85 ± 0.07	0.62 ± 0.30						

WM	DSC	HD(mm)	DSC	HD(mm)	RSD(%)	DSC	HD(mm)	RSD(%)
MD-GRU CEL	0.94 ± 0.03	0.47 ± 0.26	0.94 ± 0.02	0.51 ± 0.25	2.07 ± 2.16	0.94 ± 0.02	0.52 ± 0.22	2.40 ± 2.22
MD-GRU GDL 0.5	0.95 ± 0.02	0.43 ± 0.22	0.94 ± 0.02	0.51 ± 0.22	2.14 ± 2.35	0.94 ± 0.02	0.53 ± 0.23	2.69 ± 2.54
Manual			0.93 ± 0.02	0.54 ± 0.13	3.78 ± 3.32	0.92 ± 0.02	0.58 ± 0.15	4.59 ± 3.77
Intra-rater	0.96 ± 0.02	0.44 ± 0.15						

Finally, comparisons between GM DL 0.5, auto-weighted DL 0.5 and GDL 0.5, all with $\lambda = 0.5$, are shown in Fig. 3 on the bottom row. As can be expected, the similarity of the terms DL (1) and GDL (2) is reflected in their almost identical segmentation performance.

GM DL 0.5 shows comparable WM segmentation performance to the losses that have WM DL included. This can be explained, because the GM boundary is part of the WM boundaries and thus influences the WM scores, and furthermore the outer WM boundary is already well delineated even without any DL through the good CSF-WM contrast. Choosing a DL as a surrogate for GM DSC only, as proposed in [5], is thus justifiable.

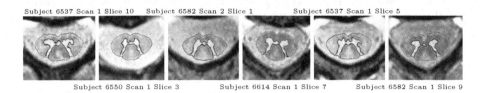

Fig. 4. Exemplary slices of the AMIRA dataset with automatic GM (*red*) and CSF-WM (*green*) boundaries, and manual GM (*blue*) and CSF-WM (*magenta*) boundaries. (Color figure online)

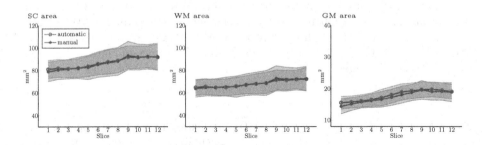

Fig. 5. SC, WM, and GM areas of GDL 0.5 (automatic) and manual segmentations wrt. the anatomical slice positions in mean ± one standard deviation.

While the SCGM challenge results only provide GM segmentation accuracy, for the AMIRA dataset we additionally also provide WM segmentation results. For the statistics, we gathered all slice-wise test results of all cross-validations for the proposed method GDL 0.5 and compare it with those of CEL. Pairwise two-tailed Hotelling's T-tests for GM accuracy in DSC and labelmap Hausdorff distance (HD) show, that the test results of the MD-GRU models trained on the different groups are not significantly different from each other ($p > 0.3$ for both GDL and CEL).

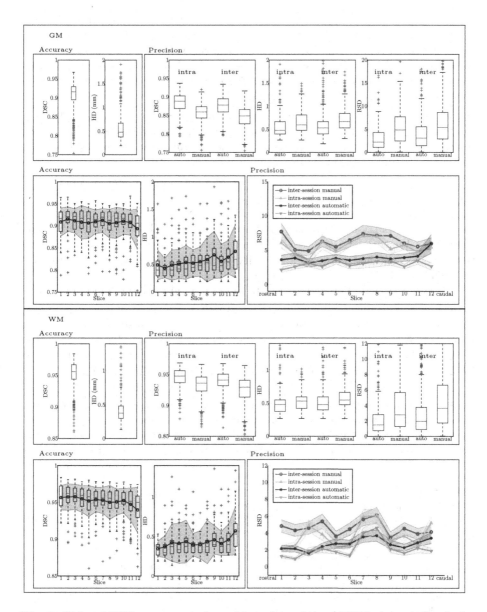

Fig. 6. GM and WM accuracy and precision plots of the AMIRA dataset. For both boxes GM and WM: *Top row:* Accuracy (*left*) in DSC and HD of all the 855 slices of the proposed method; intra-session (intra) and inter-session (inter) precision (*right*) of the proposed method (auto) and the manual segmentations in DSC, HD, and area RSD. *Bottom row:* Accuracy box plots (*left*) in DSC and HD wrt. the slice positions with overlaid error bars in the format mean ± one standard deviation; precision error bars (*right*) for area RSD wrt. the slice positions, for better visualization shown with 0.2 standard deviations. HD is measured in millimeters, and RSD in percents.

In Fig. 6 and in Table 1 we show GM and WM accuracy and precision of all gathered slice results in DSC, HD and relative standard deviation of the areas (RSD), also known as coefficient of variation. With intra- and inter-session precision we compare segmentations of the same slice for different scans with and without repositioning, respectively. The proposed automatic segmentations shows better reproducibility as the manual segmentations. Additionally, we show the anatomical GM and WM areas wrt. the slice positions in Fig. 5 and show randomly chosen results in Fig. 4. Training multiple networks with data from multiple human raters as ground truth data, as we did with the SCGM data, cf. Subsect. 4.2, might further improve the performance.

4.2   SCGM Challenge Model

To enable comparison with other methods, we tested MD-GRU on the SCGM dataset [7]. We trained four MD-GRU models, one for each expert rater's ground truth, and in the end performed majority voting on the individual test results to mimic the challenge's consensus segmentation.

We used the same MD-GRU setup but with a window size of 200×200 pixels for a similar anatomical field of view as the AMIRA models. Random subsamples in each training iteration were drawn with a distance of 200 pixels from the image boundary. We trained the networks for 100'000 iterations and observed, that the scores reached their upper bounds after around 60'000 iterations. One training iteration took around 4 s and segmentation of one slice took less than 1 s.

In Table 2, the proposed model shows a new state-of-the-art in almost all metrics. This comparison shows MD-GRU's strong performance in learning the GM segmentation problem. In Table 3, we additionally show the improvement for the auto-weighted GDL, compared to the native MD-GRU approach with only CEL. Figure 7 shows randomly chosen results of the proposed model.

Table 2. Results of the SCGM challenge competitors including the results of Porisky et al. [6], Perone et al. [5] and ours. The metrics are Dice coefficient (DSC), mean surface distance (MD), Hausdorff surface distance (HD), skeletonized Hausdorff distance (SHD), skeletonized median distance (SMD), true positive rate (TPR), true negative rate (TNR), precision (P), Jaccard index (J), and conformity (C). Best results on each metric are highlighted in bold font. Distances are measured in millimeters.

	JCSCS	DEEPSEG	MGAC	GSBME	SCT	VBEM	[6]	[5]	Proposed
DSC	0.79 ± 0.04	0.80 ± 0.06	0.75 ± 0.07	0.76 ± 0.06	0.69 ± 0.07	0.61 ± 0.13	0.80 ± 0.06	0.85 ± 0.04	$\mathbf{0.90 \pm 0.03}$
MD	0.39 ± 0.44	0.46 ± 0.48	0.70 ± 0.79	0.62 ± 0.64	0.69 ± 0.76	1.04 ± 1.14	0.53 ± 0.57	0.36 ± 0.34	$\mathbf{0.21 \pm 0.20}$
HD	2.65 ± 3.40	4.07 ± 3.27	3.56 ± 1.34	4.92 ± 3.30	3.26 ± 1.35	5.34 ± 15.35	3.69 ± 3.93	2.61 ± 2.15	$\mathbf{1.85 \pm 1.16}$
SHD	1.00 ± 0.35	1.26 ± 0.65	1.07 ± 0.37	1.86 ± 0.85	1.12 ± 0.41	2.77 ± 8.10	1.22 ± 0.51	0.85 ± 0.32	$\mathbf{0.71 \pm 0.28}$
SMD	0.37 ± 0.18	0.45 ± 0.20	0.39 ± 0.17	0.61 ± 0.35	0.39 ± 0.16	0.54 ± 0.25	0.44 ± 0.19	$\mathbf{0.36 \pm 0.17}$	0.37 ± 0.17
TPR	77.98 ± 4.88	78.89 ± 10.33	87.51 ± 6.65	75.69 ± 8.08	70.29 ± 6.76	65.66 ± 14.39	79.65 ± 9.56	94.97 ± 3.50	$\mathbf{96.22 \pm 2.69}$
TNR	$\mathbf{99.98 \pm 0.03}$	99.97 ± 0.04	99.94 ± 0.08	99.97 ± 0.05	99.95 ± 0.06	99.93 ± 0.09	99.97 ± 0.04	99.95 ± 0.06	$\mathbf{99.98 \pm 0.03}$
P	81.06 ± 5.97	82.78 ± 5.19	65.60 ± 9.01	76.26 ± 7.41	67.87 ± 8.62	59.07 ± 13.69	81.29 ± 5.30	77.29 ± 6.46	$\mathbf{85.46 \pm 4.96}$
J	0.66 ± 0.05	0.68 ± 0.08	0.60 ± 0.08	0.61 ± 0.08	0.53 ± 0.08	0.45 ± 0.13	0.67 ± 0.07	0.74 ± 0.06	$\mathbf{0.82 \pm 0.05}$
C	47.17 ± 11.87	49.52 ± 20.29	29.36 ± 29.53	33.69 ± 24.23	6.46 ± 30.59	44.25 ± 90.61	48.79 ± 18.09	64.24 ± 10.83	$\mathbf{77.46 \pm 7.31}$

Table 3. SCGM challenge results of the native MD-GRU with only CEL in comparison to the proposed GDL 0.5. Abbreviations of the metrics taken from Table 2.

	DSC	MD	HD	SHD	SMD	TPR	TNR	P	J	C
MD-GRU CEL	0.87 ± 0.03	0.30 ± 0.31	2.14 ± 1.20	0.85 ± 0.36	0.40 ± 0.20	93.93 ± 3.85	**99.98** ± 0.03	82.04 ± 5.42	0.78 ± 0.05	70.90 ± 9.06
MD-GRU GDL 0.5	**0.90** ± 0.03	**0.21** ± 0.20	**1.85** ± 1.16	**0.71** ± 0.28	**0.37** ± 0.17	**96.22** ± 2.69	**99.98** ± 0.03	**85.46** ± 4.96	**0.82** ± 0.05	**77.46** ± 7.31

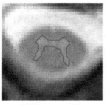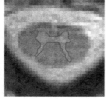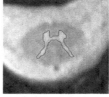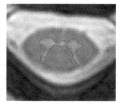

Site 1 Subject 15 Slice 2   Site 2 Subject 13 Slice 5   Site 3 Subject 12 Slice 14   Site 4 Subject 19 Slice 7

Fig. 7. For each site of the SCGM dataset, one randomly chosen result of the proposed model in cropped view.

5   Conclusion

We presented a new pipeline of acquisition and automatic segmentation of SC GM and WM. The AMIRA sequence produces 8 channel images for different inversion times which the proposed deep learning approach with MD-GRU used for segmentation. Using the 8 channels, tissue specific relaxation curves can be learned and used for GM-WM segmentation.

Comparing our segmentation results to the results of the ex-vivo high-resolution dataset of Perone et al. [5], we show comparable accuracy for in-vivo data. The acquired AMIRA dataset in scan-rescan fashion, with and without repositioning in the scanner, shows high reproducibility in terms of GM area RSD. Thus we believe that the presented pipeline is a candidate for longitudinal clinical studies. Further tests with patient data have to be conducted.

We added a generalized multi-label Dice loss to the cross entropy loss that MD-GRU uses. We observed, that the segmentation performance was stable for a larger region of the weighting λ between the two losses. In a future work, we will study the effects of small λs that correspond well with the logarithmical magnitudes of CEL. Our proposed segmentation model outperforms the methods from the SC GM segmentation challenge. Training the MD-GRU models directly on the 3D data might further improve the performance compared to slice-wise segmentation.

Given the small and fine structure of the GM, we like to point out, that the achieved results of the metrics are near optimal. Higher resolutions of the imaging sequence will improve the accuracy more easily.

Acknowledgments. We thank Dr. Matthias Weigel, Prof. Dr. Oliver Bieri and Tanja Haas for the MR acquisitions with the AMIRA sequence.

References

1. Andermatt, S., Pezold, S., Cattin, P.: Multi-dimensional gated recurrent units for the segmentation of biomedical 3D-data. In: Carneiro, G., et al. (eds.) LABELS/DLMIA-2016. LNCS, vol. 10008, pp. 142–151. Springer, Cham (2016). https://doi.org/10.1007/978-3-319-46976-8_15
2. Crum, W.R., Camara, O., Hill, D.L.G.: Generalized overlap measures for evaluation and validation in medical image analysis. IEEE Trans. Med. Imaging **25**(11), 1451–1461 (2006)
3. Datta, E., Papinutto, N., Schlaeger, R., Zhu, A., Carballido-Gamio, J., Henry, R.G.: Gray matter segmentation of the spinal cord with active contours in MR images. NeuroImage **147**, 788–799 (2017)
4. Horváth, A., et al.: A principled approach to combining inversion recovery images. In: Proceedings of the 26th Annual Meeting of ISMRM, Paris, France, June 2018
5. Perone, C.S., Calabrese, E., Cohen-Adad, J.: Spinal cord gray matter segmentation using deep dilated convolutions. Sci. Rep. **8**(1), 5966 (2018)
6. Porisky, A., et al.: Grey matter segmentation in spinal cord MRIs via 3D convolutional encoder networks with shortcut connections. In: Cardoso, M.J., et al. (eds.) DLMIA/ML-CDS-2017. LNCS, vol. 10553, pp. 330–337. Springer, Cham (2017). https://doi.org/10.1007/978-3-319-67558-9_38
7. Prados, F., et al.: Spinal cord grey matter segmentation challenge. NeuroImage **152**, 312–329 (2017)
8. Sudre, C.H., Li, W., Vercauteren, T., Ourselin, S., Jorge Cardoso, M.: Generalised dice overlap as a deep learning loss function for highly unbalanced segmentations. In: Cardoso, M.J., et al. (eds.) DLMIA/ML-CDS-2017. LNCS, vol. 10553, pp. 240–248. Springer, Cham (2017). https://doi.org/10.1007/978-3-319-67558-9_28
9. Weigel, M., Bieri, O.: Spinal cord imaging using averaged magnetization inversion recovery acquisitions. Magn. Reson. Med. **79**(4), 1870–1881 (2018)

Predicting Scoliosis in DXA Scans
Using Intermediate Representations

Amir Jamaludin[1(⊠)], Timor Kadir[2], Emma Clark[3], and Andrew Zisserman[1]

[1] VGG, Department of Engineering Science, University of Oxford, Oxford, UK
{amirj,az}@robots.ox.ac.uk
[2] Optellum, Oxford, UK
timor.kadir@optellum.com
[3] Musculoskeletal Research Unit, School of Clinical Sciences,
University of Bristol, Bristol, UK
emma.clark@bristol.ac.uk

Abstract. We describe a method to automatically predict scoliosis in Dual-energy X-ray Absorptiometry (DXA) scans. We also show that intermediate representations, which in our case are segments of body parts, help improve performance. Hence, we propose a two step process for prediction: (i) we learn to segment body parts via a segmentation Convolutional Neural Network (CNN), which we show outperforms the noisy labels it was trained on, and (ii) we predict with a classification CNN that uses as input both the raw DXA scan and also the intermediate representation, i.e. the segmented body parts. We demonstrate that this two step process can predict scoliosis with high accuracy, and can also localize the spinal curves (i.e. geometry) without additional supervision. Furthermore, we also propose a soft score of scoliosis based on the classification CNN which correlates to the severity of scoliosis.

1 Introduction

Scoliosis is an abnormal sideways curvature of the spine typically occuring prior to puberty and affects approximately 1.1% to 2.9% of children [12]. While most cases are mild, stablizing over time and presenting few symptoms, some children develop severe deformaties that can cause lifelong disability and pain. Scoliosis can also cause back pain [1] and in rare cases can cause respiratory failure [8]. It is not currently possible to determine prognosis at the onset of disease and hence children with scoliosis are monitored with repeated X-Ray imaging to determine whether the disease is stable or progressing. While accepted as the standard of care, the use of repeated X-Ray imaging on children with the associated radiation dose is far from ideal. Moreover, the radiation dose also precludes its use in population based epidemiological studies to better understand disease progression and develop future tools to predict prognosis and for screening.

DXA Scans: The use of DXA imaging for diagnosis and monitoring of scoliosis has been proposed as an alternative to X-Ray due to its very low radiation

© Springer Nature Switzerland AG 2019
G. Zheng et al. (Eds.): CSI 2018, LNCS 11397, pp. 15–28, 2019.
https://doi.org/10.1007/978-3-030-13736-6_2

dose compared to spinal X-Rays (0.001 mSv vs. 1.5 mSv) and widespread availability [12]. DXA scans, typically used to measure bone mineral density in the management of osteoporosis, are whole body scans acquired in a line scanning manner from the top of the head to the bottom of the feet. Two X-Ray sources at different energy levels are used to create a pair of absorption images which are then post-processed to produce quantitative bone mineral density images. While detection of scoliosis using DXA has been shown to be feasible and accurate, the manual technique proposed by [12] is labour intensive and requires careful adherence to the prescribed analysis protocol for accurate results. That being said, the method has proven to be quite successful in scoliosis research e.g. [5]. The technique involves first localizing important body parts to establish a reference coordinate system. These are then used for two purposes: (i) the head and legs are used to determine the overall body position because incorrect positioning can either mask or mimic the appearance of the condition, and (ii) the curvature of the spine is used to assess for the presence of the condition; defined to be when the curvature is $\geq 10°$. Our goal in this work is to automate the process of scoliosis classification using DXA, based on [12]. An overview of our approach is given in Fig. 1.

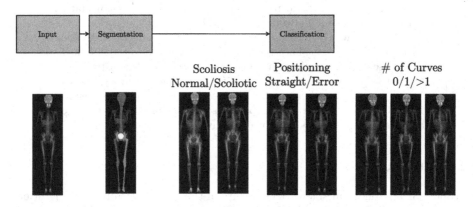

Fig. 1. Overview: a two stage approach where we take in a raw DXA scan and produces segmentation of the body parts as an intermediate step, the outputs of which are used in our classification stage.

Intermediate Representations: Our approach is based on a CNN driven by a set of intermediate representations that attempt to mimic the intuition of the underlying process of [12] described above. Our hypothesis is that such intermediate representations, in this case soft-segmentation masks, can improve classification performance, at least within the context of specific medical applications and when training with dataset sizes typically available in medical image analysis. The intermediate representations embed prior knowledge on how scoliosis is imaged and assessed in the case of DXA, and provide important cues for the network. In more detail, we provide several soft map segmentations of the key parts of the anatomy used in the DXA assessment process: the head and legs, to determine the overall body position; and the spine, so that its curvature can be used to assess for the presence and severity of the condition. In effect, the use of such intermediate representations guides the learning process to focus on important parts in determining scoliosis.

Related Work: Intermediate representations have recently been proposed as a means to extract characteristic object representations in the MarrNet 2.5D sketches by [14], and to take advantage of available training datasets for learning keypoints by [15]. Our use of intermediate representations differs from these. There has been a lot of work done on whole body DXA scans e.g. manual segmentation of body parts in [2] and modelling the shape of the body in [11]. There is also work looking at the spine using DXA, more specifically segmenting the vertebral body [9] but ours is the first system to segment the spine automatically in whole body DXA scans.

Contributions and Overview: This paper makes several contributions: (i) we present an automated method to predict scoliosis from DXA scans; (ii) we demonstrate improved classification performance of scoliosis when DXA images are augmented with application tuned intermediate representations; (iii) we illustrate how such intermediate representations may be robustly generated using a network trained on "cheaply" obtained but noisy labels; and (iv) we propose that our network can infer a continuous scale of the severity of scoliosis even though it has been trained on binary labels. The remainder of the paper is organized in two main sections: Sect. 2 describes the approach and process by which we train a (segmentation) network for generating the intermediate representations. Section 3 describes the network for predicting the scoliosis and related labels from both the DXA scans and intermediate representations. The description of the dataset and experimental results then follow in Sects. 4 and 5 respectively, including a proposal for a scoliosis score, and evidence hotspots localizing the curvature of the spine.

2   Segmentation

There are multiple body parts that can be seen in the whole body DXA scans, not all are important for predicting scoliosis. Hence, a sensible approach to automate prediction of scoliosis from these scans is to segment relevant body parts prior to classification of scoliosis. The body parts we segment are: (1) head, (2) spine, (3) pelvis, (4) pelvic cavity, (5) left leg, and (6) right leg. The spine is the most important part since scolios is a disease of the spine while the others are important for predicting positioning error (straight body vs. curved). Positioning error also plays a part in determining scoliosis as the orientation of the head and legs also affects curvature of the spine.

Since the full body DXA scans are homogeneous, segmentation labels for some parts of the body can be produced with a series of simple heuristics. These labels, although not perfect, are good enough to train a segmentation CNN and, as will be seen, in many cases the trained CNN produces visually better segmentations. In the following sections we describe the stages of training the segmentation CNN: first, generating (possibly noisy) segmentation labels using simple heuristics from classical computer vision; and second, defining loss functions and the architecture of the CNN.

2.1   Generating Segmentation Labels

For each scan, the head is first segmented via active contour around the head region [3]. The pelvis is located by scanning each row of the image starting from the bottom of the image until the bimodal intensity from the legs becomes unimodal. Working through the body in this way, using a combination of active contours and row based intensity modes, each of the body parts in turn can be segmented. Note, this is only possible because of the uniform positioning of the body adopted for the DXA scans. Around 90% of the scans are good though rough. Examples of the segmentation masks from these simple heuristics can be seen in Fig. 2.

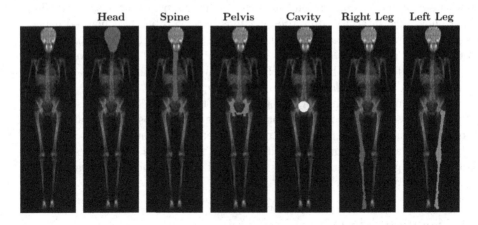

Fig. 2. Segmentation labels: the segmentation labels created by simple heuristics. Going from left to right: (1) the original image followed by segmentation masks of the (2) head, (3) spine, (4) pelvis, (5) pelvic cavity, (6) right leg, and (7) left leg.

2.2   A CNN for Segmentation

The goal is to automatically segment the labelled body parts for each DXA scan using a CNN. The segmentation CNN takes in a DXA scan as input and produces six different channels with same dimension as the input, where each channel corresponds to the six labelled parts as shown in Fig. 2. The design of the network is inspired by the U-Net architecture with minor changes [10]. The architecture of the network is given in Fig. 3.

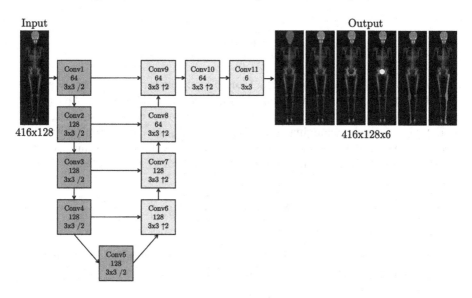

Fig. 3. Segmentation CNN: the network takes in a full body DXA scan and produces segmentation masks for each of the six body parts. The network is based on the U-Net architecture in that we have multiple skip connections from the earlier layers of the network connecting to the later layers. /2 denotes a stride of 2. The output shows the segmentation output overlaid on top of the input (in actuality the network only produces the segmentation mask).

Segmentation Losses: We consider two different losses to train the segmentation network. The first is a standard L_2 loss:

$$\mathcal{L}_{seg} = \sum_{n=1}^{N} \|y_n - \hat{y}_n\|^2 \tag{1}$$

where y_n is segmentation label (binary, $y = 1$ for parts containing a body part and $y = 0$ otherwise), and $\hat{y}_n$ is the output of the network for sample n. The loss is also balanced by the amount of background and foreground pixels in the batch during training.

Inspired by the method of which DXA scanners typically operate (similar to a line scan camera); scan line by scan line or row by row of the whole scan, we also propose a segmentation loss on a per scan line basis. This is done as follows: for each scan line, the network is tasked to predict both the mid-point and thickness of the labelled body part. The mid-point prediction can be viewed as a 128-way classification task where each class is the point of the 128-dimensional scan line (i.e. the width of the image), optimized via a standard softmax log loss:

$$\mathcal{L}_{mid} = -\sum_{n=1}^{N} \left(y_n - \log \sum_{j=1}^{128} e^{y_j(x_n)} \right) \tag{2}$$

where y_j is the jth component of the **Conv11** output for x_n per scan line. The raw output of this layer is a mid-point heatmap for each labelled body part. The prediction of thickness for each scan line can be expressed as the summation of the number of pixels belonging to a labelled body part e.g. a scan line with 8 spine pixels would have a thickness of 8 for the spine class. The same **Conv11** output y_j is used for predicting the thickness, optimized with L_2 loss:

$$\mathcal{L}_{thick} = \sum_{n=1}^{N} \left\| \sum_{j=1}^{128} y_n - \sum_{j=1}^{128} \mathcal{H}(\hat{y}_n) \right\|^2 \tag{3}$$

where $\mathcal{H}$ is the Heaviside step function which is approximated via a sigmoid, used to binarize the activation of the **Conv11** output:

$$\mathcal{H}(x) = \frac{1}{1 + e^{-k(x-0.5)}} \tag{4}$$

where k controls the steepness ($k = 10$ in our case). To produce the segmentation mask for each scan, we combine the predicted mid-point (max of the activation of **Conv11** for each scan line) and the thickness of a labelled body part for the corresponding scan line (see Fig. 4). A segmentation mask can also be produced directly after the Heaviside activation but we find this leads to be slightly worse segmentation performance.

The Benefits of Using a Segmentation CNN: Although we are able to produce segmentation masks via very simple heuristic and classical computer vision methods, in about 10% of cases there are erroneous segmentations especially for a really difficult body part like the spine. As the goal is to build an end-to-end system of scoliosis prediction, a CNN is much more suitable approach as it learns, despite the noisy training labels, to correctly predict the segmentation masks. Figure 5 shows examples of failure cases for the simple method against output of a CNN on the test set. A second benefit of using the CNN is that we obtain a 'soft-segmentation mask'. As will be seen, using this as an intermediate representation improves the classification performance compared to using the hard segmentations.

3   Classification

The goal is to predict three different classifications for each DXA scan: (i) a binary classification of scoliosis vs. non-scoliosis, outlined in [12], (ii) a binary classification of positioning error which is dependant on the straightness of the

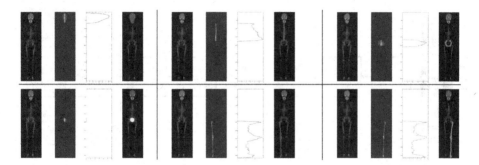

Fig. 4. Segmentation mask from mid-point and thickness: the segmentation masks from intermediate soft segmentation of the body parts, which contain mid-point information, alongside the corresponding thickness vector for each body part. We find the intermediate segmentation, or soft mask, from the raw output of **Conv11** can also be used for classifying scoliosis and other tasks.

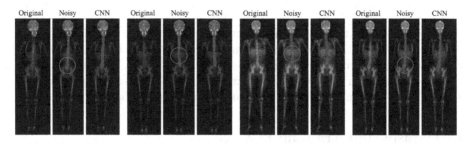

Fig. 5. Simple heuristics vs CNN: "**Noisy**" is the noisy annotation generated via simple heuristics, and used to train the CNN. We see around 10% failure cases. Here we show examples of those failure cases on the test set compared to the CNN segmentation for the spine. Failures typically appears as under-segmentation of the spine around the base or the middle of the spine highlighted in the "**Noisy**" examples.

whole body in the DXA scan, and (iii) the number of curves of a scoliotic spine (only on cases with scoliosis). The number of curves is divided into three different classes: no curve (normal spine); one curve, i.e. a "C" shaped spine; and more than one curve, which includes the classical "S" shaped spine with two curves. The networks for classification share the first six layers, five convolutional and one fully connected layer, which branch out for each of the three classification tasks (see Fig. 6).

Classification Loss: We follow the multi-task balanced loss approach discussed in [7] which can be expressed as minimizing a combination of the softmax log-losses of the three classifications:

$$\mathcal{L}_t = -\sum_{n=1}^{N} \left(y_c(x_n) - \log \sum_{j=1}^{C_t} e^{y_j(x_n)} \right) \quad (5)$$

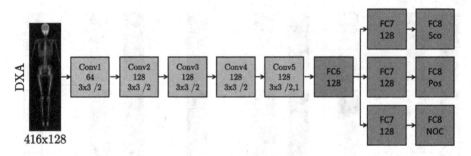

Fig. 6. Classification CNN: The network is inspired by the VGG-M network in [4] with 5 convolutional layers and 3 fully connected layers but with slightly different filter sizes and number of filters. We experimented with several different input for the classification network: (1) raw DXA scan, (2) segmentation mask, (3) mid-point map, and (4) a combination of the raw DXA and either the segmentation mask, mid-point map or both.

where t corresponds to each classification and $t \in \{1 \dots 3\}$, x is the input scan, C_t which corresponds to the number of classes in task t, y_j is the jth component of the **FC8** output, and c is the true class of x_n. The loss for each classification is also balanced with the inverse of the frequency of the class to emphasize the contribution of the minority class e.g. only 8% of the scans have scoliosis.

4   Dataset and Training Details

The dataset is from the Avon Longitudinal Study of Parents and Children (ALSPAC) cohort that recruited pregnant women in the UK. The DXA scans of the subjects were obtained from two different time points; when the subjects were 9 and 15 years of age. This difference in acquisition period and the variation of height between different individuals results in a difference of scan heights. Figure 7 shows a comparison of scans from various individuals at different time points.

In all, there are 7645 unique subjects in the dataset, most of which have two scans, which totals to 12028 scans. The distribution of labels of the different classification tasks is given in Table 1. We use a 80:10:10 (train:test:validation) random split, on a per patient basis (about 9.6k:1.2k:1.2k scans). Two different random splits of the data are used throughout (from training to evaluation) in order to obtain standard deviations on the classification performance.

Pre-processing: The scans are normalized such that both the head and feet are roughly in the same region for all the scans regardless of age and original height of the scans. Empty spaces on top of the head and below the feet are also removed. The scans are cropped isotropically to prevent distortion and to keep the aspect ratio the same as the original. The dimensions of the scans after normalization is 416×128 pixels.

9 Years Old   15 Years Old

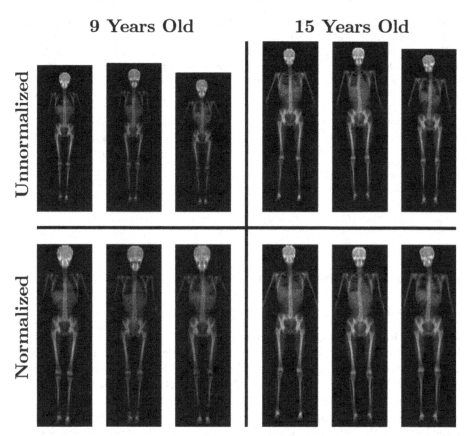

Fig. 7. Height normalization: the top row shows examples of scans prior to height normalization for both time points (9 and 15 years old), while the bottom row shows the height normalized scans.

Training Details: Both the segmentation and classification networks are optimized via stochastic gradient descent (SGD) from scratch. The hyperparameters are; batch size 64 for segmentation and 256 for classification; momentum 0.9; weight decay 0.0005; initial learning rate of 0.0001 for segmentation and 0.001 for classification, both of which are lowered by a factor of 10 as the loss plateaus. The network were trained via the MatConvNet [13] toolbox using an NVIDIA Titan X GPU. We employ several training augmentation strategies: (i) translation of ±24 pixels in the x-axis, (ii) translation of ±24 pixels in the y-axis, and (iii) random flipping. At test time, the final prediction is calculated from the average prediction of an image and its flip.

Table 1. Distribution of labels: there are three different classification tasks: (i) scoliosis, (ii) positioning, and (iii) number of curves (NOC). There are 12028 scans but fewer labels, since not all scans have labels for all three tasks.

	Normal	Abnormal	
Positioning	10139 (94.3%)	1889 (15.7%)	
Scoliosis	9435 (91.0%)	933 (9.0%)	
	0	1	>1
NOC	9435 (91.1%)	766 (7.4%)	159 (1.5%)

Table 2. The IoU of the models on the test set: "L_2" is the network trained via L_2 loss and "MT" is the network trained on minimizing the mid-point and thickness on a per scan line basis.

IoU		L_2	MT
	Head	0.93	**0.95**
	Spine	0.85	**0.87**
	Pelvis	**0.77**	0.72
	Pelvic cavity	0.64	**0.90**
	Left leg	0.80	**0.83**
	Right leg	0.81	**0.84**

5   Experiments and Results

5.1   Segmentation

Segmentation Losses Comparison: The segmentations are evaluated using the intersection over union (IoU) between the predicted output and the noisy label generated in Sect. 2.1. A CNN is trained for each loss, and their performance compared in Table 2. The performance of the network trained on the mid-point and thickness losses outperforms the network trained on the L_2 loss on every body part segmentation apart from the pelvis; 0.77 vs. 0.72. This might be due to the fact that the pelvis is a much more complex segmentation task and harder to segment on a per scan line basis. The pelvis ground truth annotations made by the simple heuristics segmentation are also a lot noisier than the other body parts.

5.2   Classification

Comparison of Input for Classification. We investigate different inputs for the CNN for predicting the three classification tasks. The different inputs are combinations of: (i) the raw DXA scan, (ii) the segmentation masks of the body parts, and (iii) a soft segmentation of the body parts obtained from the output of the **Conv11** layer from the segmentation CNN (which also has mid-point information of each body part per scan line). The network which only use the raw DXA input is considered as baseline. CNNs with multiple inputs have concatenation layers after **FC6** and share the last two layers for each task. The average per-class accuracy is given in Table 3. It can be seen that the best choices are networks that take in raw DXA together with either of the two intermediate representations, both hard and soft segmentation masks. Looking at each task individually, the best network for scoliosis is the CNN (E) that takes in both the raw DXA scan and the soft mask of the body parts, with an improvement of **+3.8%** (**86.7%** → **90.5%**) compared to the baseline CNN (A) that inputs just the raw DXA. CNN (E) outperforms the baseline by **+3.6%** (**69.0%** → **72.6%**) for predicting the number of curves. Finally, the best result for positioning error is CNN (D) which is **+0.2%** better than CNN (A) (**81.5%** → **81.7%**). To summarize, looking at Table 3, adding intermediate representation as input to the classification CNN is always better, and that when comparing intermediate representation, soft segmentation masks are better than hard (binary) segmentation masks.

Table 3. Average per-class accuracy (mean ± std %): The top three rows are the inputs used to train the network where "**Raw DXA**" is the raw DXA whole body scan, "**Mask**" is the segmentation output, binary mask of the body parts, of the segmentation CNN, and "**Soft Mask**" is the **Conv11** output of the segmentation CNN, which has both body parts localizations and mid-point information.

	A	B	C	D	E
Raw DXA	✓			✓	✓
Mask		✓		✓	
Soft Mask			✓		✓
Scoliosis	86.7 ± 2.0	82.5 ± 0.7	88.3 ± 0.1	87.3 ± 0.4	**90.5 ± 1.5**
Positioning	81.5 ± 1.8	77.6 ± 1.9	80.6 ± 1.3	**81.7 ± 0.6**	80.5 ± 0.3
$\#ofCurves$	69.0 ± 2.1	68.2 ± 8.5	70.9 ± 2.3	69.7 ± 1.2	**72.6 ± 1.2**

Classification Hotspots. We investigate the weak localization of the task learned by the CNN or evidence hotspots as in [6,7]. We follow the method outlined in [16]. The best task to look at in our case is the scoliosis prediction. Figure 8 shows different examples of scans in the test with scoliosis alongside their hotspots. As expected, the hotspots manage to localize the spines in the images, but also, interestingly, the hotspots manage to indicate which part of the spine is affected by scoliosis; in Fig. 8, we can see hotspots examples of thoracic scoliosis which localized around the thoracic region (upper spine) and examples of lumbar scoliosis which localized around the lumbar region (lower spine).

Severity of Scoliosis. The output prediction of the network, specifically scoliosis, can be interpreted as a soft score of the task (softmax of the last layer). Since the ease of predicting scoliosis directly relates to the how curved the spine

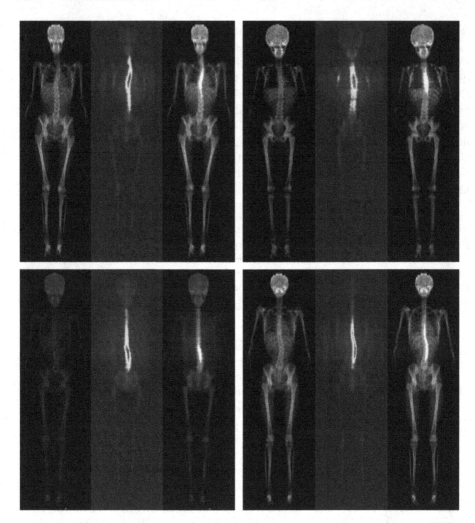

Fig. 8. Evidence hotspots of scoliosis: top row shows examples of thoracic scoliosis while bottom row shows examples of lumbar scoliosis. In each image, we show the input image, the saliency map, and the saliency map overlaid on top of the image i.e. hotspots.

is, the more confident the network is about the prediction, the more likely that the scan has scoliosis. Figure 9 shows scans on the test set alongside their soft scores. This soft score of scoliosis can be used to monitor disease progression of patients with scoliosis, where getting higher scores across a period of time i.e. a longitudinal study of the subject would mean the scoliosis is getting worse.

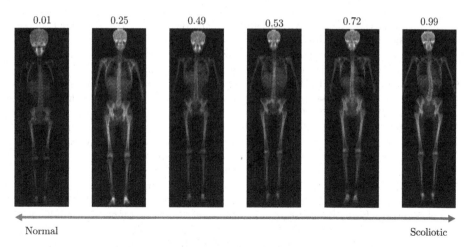

Fig. 9. Severity of scoliosis: shown are examples on the test set and their soft scores for scoliosis prediction; scans with scores approaching 1 are more scoliotic and scores approaching 0 are normal. In this example, the 3 examples on the left are normal scans and the 3 examples on the right have scoliosis.

6   Conclusion

We have shown that scoliosis can be predicted automatically via DXA scans, and that predictions can improved by adding more supervision in the form of intermediate representations, which in our case comes in the form of a soft segmentation mask of the spine and other body parts. We have also demonstrated that the evidence for the scoliosis classification can be weakly localized as hot spots, and that the score defines a grading for scoliosis severity. One possible future work is to predict the direction of the apex of the curves.

Acknowledgements. We are extremely grateful to all the families who took part in this study, the midwives for their help in recruiting them, and the whole ALSPAC team, which includes interviewers, computer and laboratory technicians, clerical workers, research scientists, volunteers, managers, receptionists and nurses. The UK Medical Research Council and the Wellcome Trust (Grant ref: 102215/2/13/2) and the University of Bristol provide core support for ALSPAC. This publication is the work of the authors and Amir Jamaludin will serve as guarantor for the contents of this paper. This research was specifically funded by the British Scoliosis Research Foundation, and the DXA scans were funded through the Wellcome Trust (grants 084632 and 079960).

References

1. Asher, M.A., Burton, D.C.: Adolescent idiopathic scoliosis: natural history and long term treatment effects. Scoliosis **1**(1), 2 (2006)
2. Burkhart, T.A., Arthurs, K.L., Andrews, D.M.: Manual segmentation of DXA scan images results in reliable upper and lower extremity soft and rigid tissue mass estimates. J. Biomech. **42**(8), 1138–1142 (2009)

3. Chan, T.F., Vese, L.A.: Active contours without edges. IEEE Trans. Image Process **10**(2), 266–277 (2001). https://doi.org/10.1109/83.902291

4. Chatfield, K., Simonyan, K., Vedaldi, A., Zisserman, A.: Return of the devil in the details: delving deep into convolutional nets. In: Proceedings of BMVC (2014)

5. Clark, E.M., Tobias, J.H., Fairbank, J.: The impact of small spinal curves in adolescents who have not presented to secondary care: a population-based cohort study. Spine **41**(10), E611–617 (2016)

6. Jamaludin, A., Kadir, T., Zisserman, A.: SpineNet: automatically pinpointing classification evidence in spinal MRIs. In: Ourselin, S., Joskowicz, L., Sabuncu, M.R., Unal, G., Wells, W. (eds.) MICCAI 2016. LNCS, vol. 9901, pp. 166–175. Springer, Cham (2016). https://doi.org/10.1007/978-3-319-46723-8_20

7. Jamaludin, A., Kadir, T., Zisserman, A.: SpineNet: automated classification and evidence visualization in spinal MRIs. Med. Image Anal. **41**, 63–73 (2017)

8. Pehrsson, K., Bake, B., Larsson, S., Nachemson, A.: Lung function in adult idiopathic scoliosis: a 20 year follow up. Thorax **46**(7), 474–478 (1991)

9. Roberts, M.G., Pacheco, E.M., Mohankumar, R., Cootes, T.F., Adams, J.E.: Detection of vertebral fractures in DXA VFA images using statistical models of appearance and a semi-automatic segmentation. Osteoporos. Int. **21**(12), 2037–2046 (2010)

10. Ronneberger, O., Fischer, P., Brox, T.: U-Net: convolutional networks for biomedical image segmentation. In: Navab, N., Hornegger, J., Wells, W.M., Frangi, A.F. (eds.) MICCAI 2015. LNCS, vol. 9351, pp. 234–241. Springer, Cham (2015). https://doi.org/10.1007/978-3-319-24574-4_28

11. Shepherd, J.A., Ng, B.K., Fan, B., Schwartz, A.V., Cawthon, P., Cummings, S.R., Kritchevsky, S., Nevitt, M., Santanasto, A., Cootes, T.F.: Modeling the shape and composition of the human body using dual energy X-ray absorptiometry images. PLoS ONE **12**(4), e0175857 (2017)

12. Taylor, H.J., et al.: Identifying scoliosis in population-based cohorts: development and validation of a novel method based on total-body dual-energy x-ray absorptiometric scans. Calcif. Tissue Int. **92**(6), 539–547 (2013)

13. Vedaldi, A., Lenc, K.: MatConvNet: convolutional neural networks for MATLAB. In: Proceedings of ACMM (2015)

14. Wu, J., Wang, Y., Xue, T., Sun, X., Freeman, W.T., Tenenbaum, J.B.: MarrNet: 3D shape reconstruction via 2.5D sketches. In: Advances in Neural Information Processing Systems (2017)

15. Wu, J., et al.: Single image 3D interpreter network. In: Leibe, B., Matas, J., Sebe, N., Welling, M. (eds.) ECCV 2016. LNCS, vol. 9910, pp. 365–382. Springer, Cham (2016). https://doi.org/10.1007/978-3-319-46466-4_22

16. Zhang, J., Bargal, S.A., Lin, Z., Brandt, J., Shen, X., Sclaroff, S.: Top-down neural attention by excitation backprop. Int. J. Comput. Vis. **126**, 1084–1102 (2017). https://doi.org/10.1007/s11263-017-1059-x

Fast Registration of CT with Intra-operative Ultrasound Images for Spine Surgery

Houssem-Eddine Gueziri[✉] and D. Louis Collins

McConnell Brain Imaging Center, Montreal Neurological Institute and Hospital,
WB221, 3801 University Street, Montreal, QC H3A 2B4, Canada
{houssem.gueziri,louis.collins}@mcgill.ca

Abstract. Intra-operative ultrasound (iUS) has a considerable potential for image-guided navigation in spinal fusion surgery. Accurate registration of pre-operative computed tomography (CT) images to the iUS images is crucial for guidance. However, low image quality and bone-related artifacts in iUS render the task challenging. This paper presents a GPU-based fast CT-to-iUS rigid registration framework of a single vertebra designed for image-guided spine surgery. First, the framework involves a straightforward iUS acquisition procedure consisting in a single sweep in the cranio-caudal axis, which allows to roughly determine the initial alignment between CT and iUS images. Then, using this as a starting point, the registration is refined by aligning the gradients that are located on the posterior surface of the vertebra to obtain the final transformation. We validated our approach on a lumbosacral section of a porcine cadaver with images from T15 to L6 vertebrae. The median target registration error was 1.48 mm (IQR = 0.68 mm), which is below the clinical acceptance threshold of 2 mm. The total registration time was $10.79\,\text{s} \pm 1.27\,\text{s}$. We believe that our approach matches the clinical needs in terms of accuracy and computation time, which makes it a potential solution to be integrated into the surgical workflow.

Keywords: Vertebra registration · Spine surgery · Ultrasound · Computed tomography · GPU

1 Introduction

Spinal fusion surgery is one of the most commonly employed procedures for treating various spinal conditions involving scoliosis, spinal stenosis, degenerative disc disease or spondylolisthesis [1]. The procedure consists in using a bone graft to fuse two or more vertebral bodies together into one single rigid structure. In most cases, the surgeon additionally uses metal plates, screws and rods to support the vertebrae while the bones fuse. A crucial part of the spinal instrumentation procedure is the placement of pedicle screws, which has been associated with high complication factors related to screw malpositioning [2]. The

© Springer Nature Switzerland AG 2019
G. Zheng et al. (Eds.): CSI 2018, LNCS 11397, pp. 29–40, 2019.
https://doi.org/10.1007/978-3-030-13736-6_3

accuracy required for pedicle screw placement varies significantly depending on the size of the screw, the vertebra level and the anatomy. Rampersaud et al. [3] reported a maximum error tolerance of screw malpositioning below 1 mm translation and 5° rotation at the midcervical spine, the midthoracic spine, and the thoracolumbar junction. The tolerance is higher in the thoracolumbar spine, where $3.8\,\text{mm}/12.7°$ at the L5 vertebra was estimated.

Image-guided navigation systems (IGNS) have been shown to reduce screw malpositioning rate by providing information on instrument localization with respect to the patient's anatomy. For IGNS to be functional during surgery, the registration step that aligns pre-operative images to the current state of the patient's anatomy must be accurate. In a standard clinical procedure, the registration is achieved by manually identifying homologous anatomical landmarks on both the pre-operative images and the patient. The procedure lasts approximately 10 to 15 min for each vertebra [4,5]. This approach is tedious, extends the operating time and is subject to operator variability. Moreover, during navigation, a dynamic reference object (DRO) (i.e., a spatially tracked tool) is rigidly attached to the spinous process of a vertebra and serves as a reference coordinate frame to account for patient positioning and motion during surgery. Once the registration achieved, changes in the position of the DRO caused by patient movement, surgical interventions or inadvertent contact with the DRO, may invalidate the registration.

Common commercial IGNS, such as the O-arm (Medtronic inc., Minneapolis, MN), Airo Mobile (Brainlab, Feldkirchen, Germany), SpineMask (Stryker, Kalamazoo, MI) or Ziehm Vision FD Vario 3D (Ziehm Imaging, Orlando, FL) use fluoroscopy or computed tomography (CT) intra-operative imaging. The latter imaging modalities introduce risks of harmful radiation exposure for both the patient and the operating room (OR) personnel. Moreover, they require a typical setup time of ~15 min [6] and extra personnel for manipulating the equipment, which significantly extends the surgical procedure time.

Intra-operative ultrasound (iUS) has been investigated as possible alternative imaging in orthopedic and spine surgery applications [7–9]. With low cost, non-ionizing radiation exposure, small footprint and a significantly shorter setup time in the OR, iUS imaging is a good candidate for image-guided navigation. However, ultrasound images can have low image quality affecting the registration accuracy, a limited field of view precluding imaging large or distant structures, and shadow artifacts induced by high acoustic absorption of bones, which hinder their application in clinical environment.

The goal of this paper is to propose an OR-designed fast CT-to-iUS image registration method for spine surgery. Specifically, we present a *rigid registration* framework to align pre-operative CT to iUS images of a *single vertebra*. Considering the rigid anatomical structure of the bones, single vertebra registration is a common step to achieve a more global group-wise multi-vertebrae registration to capture the spine curvature [10–12]. The motivations behind this work are three-fold: (i) to develop a radiation-free approach that relies solely on iUS imaging, (ii) to design an unobtrusive and straightforward procedure compatible with the surgical workflow, and (iii) to design a fast registration method that allows the surgeon to rapidly realign the images to correct for patient-to-image misregistration during surgery. The remainder of this paper is organized as follows: Sect. 2 reviews previous work using iUS-based IGNS in spine surgery. Section 3 presents the proposed registration framework. The experimentation setup is described in Sect. 4 and results are presented in Sect. 5.

2   Related Work

In order to achieve high CT-to-iUS registration accuracy, several authors have exploited unique properties of iUS imaging. Strong ultrasound reflections on bone structures cause the vertebra to appear in black on iUS images with a hyper echoic edge several mm thick on the bone surface [13]. Yan et al. [4,14] proposed to use a *backward* and a *forward* tracing approaches to first extract the posterior surface of the vertebra on both iUS and CT images, respectively. Then, a rigid cross-correlation registration is applied to align the vertebra surfaces. Authors reported a median target registration error (TRE) ranging between 1.65–2.31 mm on porcine cadavers. A slice-to-volume variant of the approach proposed in [15], in which the registration is performed without iUS volume reconstruction to accelerate the computations, achieved comparable accuracy. The reported registration time was around 120 s per vertebra. Both methods require an initial alignment, assumed to be achieved prior to the registration with a landmark-based manual registration.

A hierarchical CT-to-iUS vertebra registration framework was proposed by Koo et al. [8]. The registration involves three steps. First, similar to Yan's approach [4], a landmark-based manual registration is applied for an initial guess of the alignment, followed by a rigid cross-correlation registration of the posterior vertebral surface extracted on both iUS and CT imaging. The vertebra surfaces are extracted with the backward and forward tracing methods. Finally, an additional intensity-based rigid registration is performed between the vertebra surface on the CT image and the original iUS image. The average TRE reported was 2.18 mm ± 0.82 mm (ranging between 0.89–4.45 mm) on a porcine cadaver. Excluding the manual landmark registration, intensity-based registrations were achieved in ∼100 s per vertebra.

Nagpal et al. [10] proposed a multi-vertebrae CT-to-iUS registration framework. Here again, the posterior surface of the vertebrae is exploited [16] and the registration is achieved in three steps. First, with the assumption that both CT and iUS images represent similar structures, the initial alignment is obtained by applying a rigid registration using mutual information on the vertebra surface images. Then, the registration is refined by applying a global point-based registration using the vertebra surface coordinate points. To account for the spine curvature over multiple vertebrae, an additional group-wise vertebra registration is performed, in which intervertebral points are manually added to prevent physically incoherent transformations. Because, the study was conducted on clinical data of human subjects, a gold standard registration was not possible,

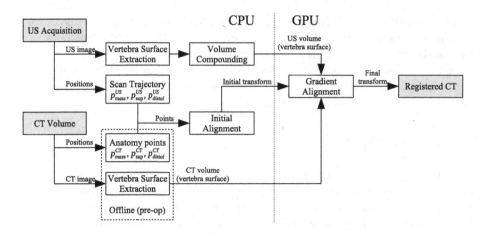

Fig. 1. Flowchart of the proposed registration framework.

authors used manual landmark registration combined with the proposed method to serve as ground truth registration. They reported average TRE of anatomical landmarks ranging from 0.71–1.70 mm and a computation time ranging from 50–185 s.

3   Registration Framework

Figure 1 shows an overview of the proposed registration framework. The approach involves four intra-operative steps: (1) extract the posterior surface of the vertebra on iUS images, (2) create an iUS compounded volume from iUS acquisition slices, (3) estimate the initial alignment, and (4) perform gradient alignment of the vertebra surfaces of CT and iUS images. The posterior vertebra surfaces on CT and iUS images are extracted using the forward and backward tracing methods [4]. The approach has the advantage to be fast and provides good results.

3.1   Intra-operative Ultrasound Image Acquisition

We use an iUS-based navigation system composed of an optical tracking camera (Polaris, Northern Digital Inc., Ontario, Canada), an ultrasound machine with a tracked phased array probe (HDI 5000/P4-7, Philips, Amsterdam, Netherlands) and a tracked tool used as a DRO. The ultrasound probe is calibrated such that collected images are associated with their respective spatial position and orientation relative to the DRO. The *Intraoperative Brain Imaging System* (IBIS) [17] open-source plate-form is used for navigation, i.e., probe calibration, tracking and 3D visualization.

The acquisition frame rate of iUS images is around 25 Hz, which may introduce redundant information in successive frames. To reduce the computation

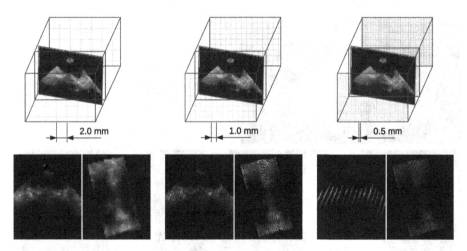

Fig. 2. Examples of ultrasound volume compounding with a resolution of $2 \times 2 \times 2\,\mathrm{mm}^3$ (left), $1 \times 1 \times 1\,\mathrm{mm}^3$ (middle) and $0.5 \times 0.5 \times 0.5\,\mathrm{mm}^3$ (right).

time of vertebra surface extraction and volume compounding, the number of acquired frames is reduced such as a minimum distance $d \in \mathbb{R}_{\geq 0}$ separates the centroids of successive frames. A high value of d yields a sparse volume and fast computations, while a value of zero does not modify the acquisition. The frames satisfying the distance criterion are selected for the next steps.

3.2 Ultrasound Volume Compounding

The selected frames are combined into a single volume by aggregating the ultrasound slices to form a resampled volume, the *compounded volume*, to avoid a full volume reconstruction as proposed in [15]. Because the relationship between the spatial positions of the ultrasound slices is fixed, registering the compounded volume to the CT volume is analogous to simultaneously optimizing for a slice-to-volume rigid body registration of each individual iUS slice to the CT volume. In our implementation, each iUS pixel intensity is resampled in its corresponding 3D location in the compounded volume, and the intensities are averaged for overlapping pixels. It is important to consider the spatial resolution of the resampled compounded volume. Figure 2 shows examples of volume compounding with different resolutions. While a fine resolution results in a large but highly sparse volume, a coarse resolution results in a small but dense volume. Note that because we use gradient information in the final alignment step, a too sparse volume precludes capturing inter-slice gradient information.

3.3 Initial Alignment

In order to guess the initial alignment, we define a simple sweep procedure to limit the variability in the translational and angular positioning of the iUS

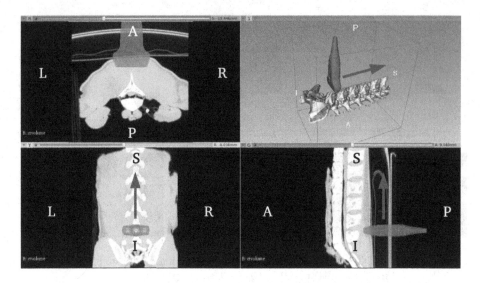

Fig. 3. Illustration of the acquisition procedure.

probe during the acquisition. The quality of the iUS acquisition has a significant impact on the registration [14]. Thus, our acquisition procedure consists in a single axial sweep along the cranio-caudal direction, starting from the inferior extremity up to the superior extremity of the vertebra, with the probe orientation normal to the coronal plane (Fig. 3).

This acquisition procedure has three key properties: (1) assuming that the same number of vertebrae is imaged with both CT and iUS, the center of mass of the selected iUS frame centroids roughly correspond to the center of the CT image, (2) the scan trajectory is approximately linear along the inferior to superior axis, (3) on the iUS image plane, the proximal to distal axis from the probe's transducers corresponds to the posterior to anterior axis on the vertebra. Based on this, three anatomical points are created on the physical space: a center of mass $\mathbf{p}_{mass}^{US}$, a superior point $\mathbf{p}_{sup}^{US}$ at a 10 mm distance from $\mathbf{p}_{mass}^{US}$ toward the superior direction, and a distal point $\mathbf{p}_{distal}^{US}$ at a 10 mm distance from $\mathbf{p}_{mass}^{US}$ toward the anterior direction. Similarly, three homologous points $\mathbf{p}_{mass}^{CT}$, $\mathbf{p}_{sup}^{CT}$ and $\mathbf{p}_{distal}^{CT}$ are created on the CT image. Finally, the initial alignment transform is obtained by applying a Procrustes point-based rigid registration, minimizing the least-square distances between the CT and the iUS points.

3.4   GPU-Based Gradient Alignment Registration

The initial alignment approach roughly registers the CT to iUS images, based on the acquisition procedure described in Sect. 3.3. To refine the registration, we perform a gradient alignment registration [18]. Originally, the approach was designed for brain MR-to-iUS registration. First, the gradient from both the fixed iUS image and the moving CT image are extracted. Then, a covariance matrix adaptation (CMA) evolution strategy [19] is used to maximize the inner product of the normalized gradients:

$$S(\nabla I_{\mathrm{US}}(\mathbf{x}), \nabla I_{\mathrm{CT}}(\mathbf{x})) = \left\langle \frac{\nabla I_{\mathrm{US}}(\mathbf{x})}{|\nabla I_{\mathrm{US}}(\mathbf{x})|}, \frac{\nabla I_{\mathrm{CT}}(\mathbf{x})}{|\nabla I_{\mathrm{CT}}(\mathbf{x})|} \right\rangle^n, \tag{1}$$

where $\mathbf{x}$ is the image coordinate vector, ∇I_{US} and ∇I_{CT} are the fixed iUS and moving CT image gradients, respectively, and $n \in \mathbb{N}$ is a free parameter which characterizes the matching criterion and was set to $n = 64$. To reduce the computation time, the metric is computed on a subset of points sampled among the most confident gradients on the image. We slightly modified the algorithm to take into account the vertebra surface on the intra-operative images. Instead of a random sampling over the entire image, the points are sampled from a 2 mm thick region around the iUS extracted bone surface. Candidates satisfying the low uncertainty criterion (see [18] for details) *among the bone surface points* are then selected to be used in Eq. (1). Gradient image computations of ∇I_{US} and ∇I_{CT}, and evaluation of the similarity metric in Eq. (1) are performed on a GPU. The final registration transform is given by:

$$T^{\mathrm{reg}} = \arg \max_T S\Big(\nabla I_{\mathrm{US}}(\mathbf{x}), \nabla I_{\mathrm{CT}}(T(\mathbf{x}))\Big). \tag{2}$$

Finally, we perform the registration using a multi-scale approach. Two different scales are used. In the first pass, the images are smoothed using a Gaussian filter with $\sigma = 2$ mm to capture large structures, e.g., thicker surface of the vertebra. A second registration pass is then performed on images filtered with $\sigma = 1$ mm.

4 Experiments

We validated our proposed registration framework on the same dataset used in [14]. The dataset contains a CT scan of a lumbosacral section of a porcine cadaver in supine position, in which vertebrae T15 and L1 to L6 were present. The CT scan consists in a superior to inferior axial slices acquired using a Picker International PQ6000 CT scanner with an in-slice resolution of 0.35×0.35 mm^2 and a slice thickness of 2 mm.

For each vertebra, three to four fiducials were implanted on the anterior/ventral part of the cadaver, such that they do not interfere with the iUS acquisition. The fiducials are made of pipette tips that can be nested together. Each fiducial is composed of three parts: a *fiducial base* which is rigidly fixed to the vertebra, an *imaging marker* which is a steel sphere inside the pipette that appears bright in CT images, and a *reference marker* which is a filled pipette such that its center corresponds to the center of the sphere in the imaging marker. Imaging fiducial positions were collected by computing the centers of the segmented bright spheres that appear on the CT image. Reference fiducial positions were manually collected using a tracked pointer with IBIS. The ground truth registration transform of each vertebra was obtained by applying a point-based registration on its corresponding fiducials.

The fiducials were used to establish the ground truth registration transform. Therefore, using the fiducial positions to assess vertebrae alignment is not suitable. In fact, computing the fiducial registration error (FRE) may not be representative of the TRE at the vertebra surface. Moreover, because the fiducials were placed far from the vertebra surface, a small misalignment of the fiducial points (i.e., small FRE) may result in a large TRE at the vertebra surface. To evaluate the TRE of the registration, seven landmarks were manually identified on the surface of each vertebra on the CT images. The anatomical landmarks correspond to: a point on the apex of the spinous process, two points on the left and right laminae, two points on the left and right superior articular processes and two points on the left and right inferior articular processes. The TRE of each vertebra is obtained by:

$$TRE_v = \sqrt{\frac{1}{7} \sum_i^7 |T^{gt}\mathbf{p}_i - T^{reg}\mathbf{p}_i|^2}, \tag{3}$$

where v is the vertebra level, T^{gt} is the ground truth registration transform obtained from fiducial point-based registration and $\mathbf{p}_i$ is the ith landmark point manually positioned on the vertebra surface. In the literature [10,14], a threshold of 2 mm is commonly used to characterize a successful registration, i.e., the registration is considered successful if its associated TRE is below 2 mm. Similarly, in our experiment, we use a 2 mm threshold to report the success rate of the registration.

In addition to the registration accuracy, we measured the computation time required to perform the registration of each vertebra. The computations involve three main tasks: extracting the vertebra surface (backward tracing), compounding the iUS volume and aligning CT to iUS volumes (i.e., solving Eq. (2)). We also report the computation time required to perform the initial alignment, although it can be neglected due to its small contribution to the overall registration time. Note that the iUS acquisition time, i.e., the time required to manipulate the iUS probe and perform the sweep, is not reported in this study. All computations were performed using an Intel© Core™ i7-3820 CPU at 3.6 GHz × 8 station and a NVIDIA GeForce GTX 670 graphics card with 4 Gb of memory.

Using a stochastic CMA evolution strategy to optimize Eq. (2) yields non-deterministic results. To measure the overall registration accuracy, for each vertebra, 10 batches of registrations are performed. Each batch involves two steps. The first step, referred to as *Reconstruction*, consists in performing a vertebra surface extraction on the iUS image and a slice compounding into a volume. The second step, referred to as *Registration*, consists in performing 10 repetitions of the CT-to-iUS registration, i.e., an initial alignment followed by a gradient alignment. In total, 100 registration trials where performed for each vertebra. It should be noted that the trials use the same CT and iUS acquisition images for each vertebra. We set the distance threshold for acquisition frame reduction $d = 0.5$ mm (see Sect. 3.1). The resolution of the iUS compounded volume (see Sect. 3.2) is set to $1.5 \times 1.5 \times 1.5$ mm^3, to produce sufficiently dense volumes.

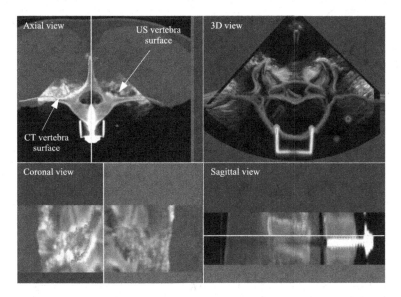

Fig. 4. Example of qualitative results showing superimposition of a registered CT image and a iUS image of the L4 vertebra: (red) iUS image, (blue) vertebra surface extracted on iUS with backward tracing, (gray) CT image, (green) vertebra surface extracted on CT with forward tracing. (Color Figure online)

5 Results

Figure 4 shows a qualitative result obtained with the proposed registration framework and the quantitative accuracy results are summarized in Table 1. The overall TRE is slightly better than the results reported in [14] with the inferior to superior axial iUS acquisition scan (ultrasound sweep No. 1). The median TRE is 1.48 mm (IQR 0.68 mm) ranging from 0.45 mm to 2.78 mm, which is below the acceptance threshold of 2 mm. This is highlighted by a success rate of 84.42%. However, the results obtained on the L4 vertebra seem to be the worst, with a median TRE of 2.03 mm. The reason behind this large error may be related to the large FRE of 0.593 mm induced when the ground truth registration was generated at L4.

The number of selected frames and the computation time for each vertebra registration are summarized in Table 2. The average overall registration time is 0.742 s ± 0.037 s per vertebra. This includes both the initial alignment and the gradient alignment processing time. This is significantly lower than the 2 min reported by Yan et al. [15] and the 100 s reported by Koo et al. [8] per each vertebra registration. The registration time ranging between 50–185 s reported by Nagpal et al. [10] involved multiple vertebrae registration, precluding a direct comparison. It should be noted that all the aforementioned works did not include the iUS volume reconstruction time, which is expected to be performed after acquiring the iUS images during the surgery. In our approach, the computational

Table 1. Registration accuracy results for each vertebra level: (left) target registration error (TRE) after the initial alignment, (middle left) TRE after final registration, (middle right) success rate below 2 mm, and (right) fiducial registration error of the ground truth registration.

Vertebra level	Initial alignment TRE (mm)	Final TRE (mm)			Success rate (%)	FRE (mm)
		Median	IQR	Range		
T15	3.714	1.20	0.30	[0.60, 1.88]	100	0.303
L1	2.916	0.84	0.32	[0.45, 1.39]	100	0.197
L2	2.439	1.37	0.44	[0.61, 2.21]	95	0.27
L3	3.698	1.40	0.32	[0.83, 2.21]	98	0.257
L4	5.916	2.03	0.35	[1.36, 2.78]	47	0.593
L5	8.32	1.69	0.42	[0.95, 2.47]	79	0.359
L6	9.185	1.75	0.46	[1.09, 2.66]	72	0.321
All vertebrae		1.48	0.68		84.42	0.328
Yan et al. [14]		1.93	0.72			

Table 2. Computation time results: GPU computations are indicated by a *.

Vertebra level	Frames		Computation time (s)				Total
	Total	Selected	Reconstruction		Registration		
			Surface extraction	Volume compounding	Initial alignment	Gradient alignment*	
T15	197	106 (53%)	8.00	4.93	0.044	0.736	13.72
L1	209	80 (38%)	6.04	3.81	0.045	0.667	10.56
L2	219	83 (37%)	6.26	4.12	0.045	0.695	11.12
L3	215	76 (35%)	5.75	3.58	0.044	0.680	10.06
L4	205	79 (38%)	5.92	3.59	0.045	0.707	10.26
L5	211	81 (38%)	6.09	3.54	0.046	0.702	10.38
L6	235	76 (32%)	5.70	3.04	0.046	0.693	9.48
Average	–	–	6.25	3.80	0.045	0.69	10.79

bottleneck is associated with the reconstruction step with an average time of $10.05\,\mathrm{s} \pm 1.26\,\mathrm{s}$. This is expected since the reconstruction task is performed on a CPU. Including the reconstruction and the registration, the total time to align the pre-operative CT image to the iUS image is $10.79\,\mathrm{s} \pm 1.27\,\mathrm{s}$, which is practical in the OR. Reducing the number of acquisition frames allows to reduce the reconstruction time. Particularly for the vertebra surface extraction step where the computation time corresponds to ~58% of the overall registration time.

6   Conclusion

In this paper, we presented a registration framework to rigidly align a CT volume to iUS images of a single vertebra. We demonstrated that our approach can achieve a median accuracy of 1.48 mm ranging from 0.45 mm to 2.78 mm on a lumbosacral section of a porcine cadaver. This is below the clinical acceptance threshold of 2 mm suggested in the literature. More importantly, with a straightforward iUS acquisition procedure and a highly efficient computation time of ~11 s, the registration framework can be easily integrated into the surgical workflow. We estimate the entire registration procedure (including the iUS acquisition) to be completed in less than one minute, rather than the 15 min required using an intra-operative CT imaging system. This allows fast corrections of registration misalignment during the surgery, without additional exposure to radiation.

Future work will involve an extended validation of the registration framework. Because the quality of the iUS acquisition may have a significant impact on the registration outcome [14], we will analyze how violation of the proposed iUS acquisition procedure affects the registration results. We will also investigate efficient methods to perform the reconstruction step on a GPU. In fact, parallelizing the extraction of the vertebra surface and the iUS volume compounding will result in further gain in computation time.

References

1. Rajaee, S.S., Bae, H.W., Kanim, L.E., Delamarter, R.B.: Spinal fusion in the united states: analysis of trends from 1998 to 2008. Spine **37**(1), 67–76 (2012)
2. Su, A.W., Habermann, E.B., Thomsen, K.M., Milbrandt, T.A., Nassr, A., Larson, A.N.: Risk factors for 30-Day unplanned readmission and major perioperative complications after spine fusion surgery in adults: a review of the national surgical quality improvement program database. Spine **41**(19), 1523–1534 (2016)
3. Rampersaud, Y.R., Simon, D.A., Foley, K.T.: Accuracy requirements for image-guided spinal pedicle screw placement. Spine **26**(4), 352–359 (2001)
4. Yan, C.X., Goulet, B., Pelletier, J., Chen, S.J.S., Tampieri, D., Collins, D.L.: Towards accurate, robust and practical ultrasound-CT registration of vertebrae for image-guided spine surgery. Int. J. Comput. Assist. Radiol. Surg. **6**(4), 523–537 (2011)
5. Arand, M., Hartwig, E., Kinzl, L., Gebhard, F.: Spinal navigation in tumor surgery of the thoracic spine: first clinical results. Clin. Orthop. Relat. Res. **399**, 211–218 (2002)
6. Scheufler, K.M., Franke, J., Eckardt, A., Dohmen, H.: Accuracy of image-guided pedicle screw placement using intraoperative computed tomography-based navigation with automated referencing, part I: cervicothoracic spine. Neurosurgery **69**(4), 782–795 (2011)
7. Hacihaliloglu, I., Abugharbieh, R., Hodgson, A.J., Rohling, R.N.: Bone surface localization in ultrasound using image phase-based features. Ultrasound Med. Biol. **35**(9), 1475–1487 (2009)

8. Koo, T.K., Kwok, W.E.: Hierarchical CT to ultrasound registration of the lumbar spine: a comparison with other registration methods. Ann. Biomed. Eng. **44**(10), 2887–2900 (2016)

9. Wein, W., Karamalis, A., Baumgartner, A., Navab, N.: Automatic bone detection and soft tissue aware ultrasound-CT registration for computer-aided orthopedic surgery. Int. J. Comput. Assist. Radiol. Surg. **10**(6), 971–979 (2015)

10. Nagpal, S., et al.: A multi-vertebrae CT to US registration of the lumbar spine in clinical data. Int. J. Comput. Assist. Radiol. Surg. **10**(9), 1371–1381 (2015)

11. Gill, S., et al.: Biomechanically constrained groupwise ultrasound to CT registration of the lumbar spine. Med. Image Anal. **16**(3), 662–674 (2012)

12. Reaungamornrat, S., Wang, A.S., Uneri, A., Otake, Y., Khanna, A.J., Siewerdsen, J.H.: Deformable image registration with local rigidity constraints for cone-beam CT-guided spine surgery. Phys. Med. Biol. **59**(14), 3761–3787 (2014)

13. Hacihaliloglu, I.: Ultrasound imaging and segmentation of bone surfaces: a review. Technology **05**(02), 74–80 (2017)

14. Yan, C.X.B., Goulet, B., Chen, S.J.S., Tampieri, D., Collins, D.L.: Validation of automated ultrasound-CT registration of vertebrae. Int. J. Comput. Assist. Radiol. Surg. **7**(4), 601–610 (2012)

15. Yan, C.X., Goulet, B., Tampieri, D., Collins, D.L.: Ultrasound-CT registration of vertebrae without reconstruction. Int. J. Comput. Assist. Radiol. Surg. **7**(6), 901–909 (2012)

16. Foroughi, P., Boctor, E., Swartz, M.J., Taylor, R.H., Fichtinger, G.: Ultrasound bone segmentation using dynamic programming. In: IEEE Ultrasonics Symposium Proceedings, pp. 2523–2526 (2007)

17. Drouin, S., et al.: IBIS: an OR ready open-source platform for image-guided neurosurgery. Int. J. Comput. Assist. Radiol. Surg. **12**(3), 363–378 (2017)

18. De Nigris, D., Collins, D.L., Arbel, T.: Fast rigid registration of pre-operative magnetic resonance images to intra-operative ultrasound for neurosurgery based on high confidence gradient orientations. Int. J. Comput. Assist. Radiol. Surg. **8**(4), 649–661 (2013)

19. Hansen, N., Ostermeier, A.: Completely derandomized self-adaptation in evolution strategies. Evol. Comput. **9**(2), 159–195 (2001)

Automated Grading of Modic Changes Using CNNs – Improving the Performance with Mixup

Dimitrios Damopoulos[1]($\boxtimes$), Daniel Haschtmann[2], Tamás F. Fekete[2], and Guoyan Zheng[1]

[1] Institute for Surgical Technology and Biomechanics,
University of Bern, Bern, Switzerland
dimitrios.damopoulos@istb.unibe.ch
[2] Schulthess Clinic, Spine Center, Zürich, Switzerland

Abstract. We propose a method for automated grading of the vertebral end-plate regions according to the Modic changes scale based on the VGG16 network architecture. We evaluate four variations of the method in a standard 9-fold cross-validation study setup on a heterogeneous dataset of 92 cases. Due to the very weak representation of the Modic Type III in the dataset, we focus on the grading of Modic Type I and Modic Type II. Despite the relatively small size of our dataset, the pipeline demonstrated a performance that is similar to or better than those achieved by the state-of-the-art methods. In particular, the most performant variant achieved an accuracy of 88.0% with an average-per-class accuracy of 77.3%. When the method is used as a binary detector for the presence or not of Modic changes, the achieved average-per-class accuracy is 92.3%. Our evaluation also suggests that the so-called mixup strategy is particularly useful for this type of classification task.

Keywords: Modic changes · Automated grading · Mixup · VGG

1 Introduction

The term *Modic changes* (MCs) refers to specific patterns of intensity variation in the signal of the T1 and T2 MR scans of the spine, occurring in the bone marrow region around the vertebral endplates. They were first mentioned in 1987 [1] and they are then named after the first author of [2, 3], where three types of such patterns were defined and their possible association with degenerative disk disease (DDD) was discussed.

Specifically, a *Type I Modic change* is defined as the presence of a bone morrow region which has a lower intensity than its surrounding tissue in a T1 scan and a higher intensity in a T2 scan, indicating a bone marrow oedema. In a *Type II Modic change*, the intensity of the region is higher than its surrounding tissue in both the T1 and T2 scans, indicating local fatty degeneration. Finally, in *Type III Modic change* the intensity is lower in both the T1 and T2 scans, representing sclerotic changes of the endplates that result in low signal in both sequences. For brevity, we will refer to these grades as *MC-I*, *MC-II* and *MC-III* respectively. Figure 1 shows a representative example for MC-I and MC-II from the dataset of our study.

© Springer Nature Switzerland AG 2019
G. Zheng et al. (Eds.): CSI 2018, LNCS 11397, pp. 41–52, 2019.
https://doi.org/10.1007/978-3-030-13736-6_4

MCs are considered to be clinically important, especially MC-I and MC-II. There has been evidence suggesting a correlation between the presence of these two MC types (especially MC-I) and low back pain (LBP) [2, 4–7], however the etiology of the MCs and how they are linked to either LBP or DDD remains an active research topic [4, 9]. Research related to MCs is complicated by the subjectability of the MC grading to inter-rater disagreement [10]. The variability in grading can be reduced substantially if the grading process is more strictly standardized and when the raters get more experienced in the task [4, 8, 10]. However, both of these conditions need time to be satisfied. Moreover, grading every case manually on a large dataset is a time-consuming process.

In this study, we propose a pipeline for the automated grading of the endplate regions around the intervertebral disks (IVDs) of the lumbar spine according the MC scale. As a component of a computer aided diagnosis system, we envision that such a method can be useful in a clinical setting by automatically pinpointing IVD regions in an MRI which might require further attention by the clinician, as possible sources of LBP. Furthermore, it can facilitate the conduction of large population studies related to MCs, as it can minimize the tedious task of annotating manually the large number of cases typically stored in a PACS system.

Despite the small size of the dataset that was used, we were able to achieve a MC-detection rate which is on par with the reported performances of human raters. A highlight of the presented work is the application of the mixup strategy [16], which we found to be effective for this particular type of classification task. In particular, we make the following contributions:

(a) We present a learning-based method for the automated grading of MCs, reporting an accuracy which is better than that of the other published work on this task [12]. The dataset that was available in the present study consisted of 92 cases, as opposed to 388 of [12].

(b) We present a successful application of the mixup strategy as introduced in [16] for data augmentation. Mixup appears to be well-suited for this problem, assisting us in coping with the inherent imbalance of this classification task.

1.1 Related Work

A method for the automated detection of MCs was first proposed in [11], which requires the manual segmentation of the IVDs, it consults only one T2 slice for the detection and it performs only binary classification (presence or not of a MC). The first complete system for automatic MC grading was proposed in [12], which also includes an automatic module for the localization of the vertebrae and their corners, making the whole pipeline fully automatic. Their proposed system achieved a 87.8% classification accuracy. The same authors proposed a multi-task CNN architecture in [14], yielding impressive performance in a variety of spine-related computer-aided diagnosis tasks. One of them was the detection of bone marrow defects of the upper and lower vertebrae of IVD regions, which they were able to detect with an accuracy of 91.0% and 90.3% respectively with their best performing models, approaching their intra-rater accuracy. These defects appear to be very similar to MCs, however they are not the same, since they are graded after consulting T2 slices only. The datasets used in the latter two works were rather extensive, consisting of the annotated scans of 388 patients in the case of [12] and of 2009 patients in the case of [14].

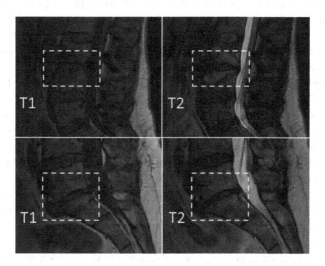

Fig. 1. Two characteristic cases of MCs from the dataset of the present study. The top T1 and T2 slices depict a MC-I case at level L3/L4 and the bottom a MC-II case at level L5/S1. The affected regions are highlighted with yellow rectangles. For the case of MC-I, the affected bone marrow region is visibly hypointense on T1 and hyperintense on T2, whereas the for the MC-II case the bone marrow is hyperintense on both modalities. (Color figure online)

2   Method

The aim of the present study is to automatically grade a given pair of T1 and T2 sequences of regions of interest that capture the upper and lower marrow regions around a particular IVD according to the MC grading system. We will refer to the two sequences of regions of interest as *IVD volumes* and to their individual slices are *IVD regions*. We restrict our attention to the following six spinal levels: T12/L1, L1/L2, L2/L3, L3/L4, L4/L5 and L5/S1. For the rest of the discussion, we will refer to these as *IVD levels*. Example IVD volumes are illustrated in Fig. 2.

As mentioned earlier, there are three MC types defined. However, in the dataset that was utilized in this study, the number of cases with MC-III was very limited. Due to this limitation and also because of the limited clinical significance of MC-III, it was decided to restrict the set of the grades to the first two types, i.e. MC I and MC II. For convenience, we will also refer to the absence of any MC on some IVD level as *MC-0* (background class). Thus, there are $M = 3$ classes in total, MC-0, MC-I and MC-II.

2.1 Isolation of the IVD Regions

The input to the pipeline is a sequence of T1-weighed and a sequence of T2-weighted sagittal MR scans of a lumbar spine. Additionally, it is assumed that a prior localization step has taken place that can provide estimations for the centers of the depicted IVDs, their orientations and their widths. We are interested only in the projection of these elements on the sagittal plane, therefore, for each IVD, we assume the availability of: (a) its 2D center on the sagittal plane and (b) a 2D vector, whose angular displacement represents its orientation and its length is equal to the width of the IVD.

The supplied information is utilized for the extraction of rectangular IVD regions. The extracted IVD regions are centered around their corresponding 2D IVD center, they are parallel to the identified orientation and their size is proportional to the identified width, with their aspect ratio set to 2:1. For the extraction of the IVD volume, this operation is carried out on five of the slices of the input T1 sequence and five of these slices of the input T2 sequence, symmetrically around their midsagittal slice. The same center, orientation and width are used for the extraction of all the 10 IVD regions of the two IVD volumes. In [12], a rigid registration step was also employed for the extraction of the IVD regions in order to account for the small possible movement of the patient between the acquisition of the two sequences. In the present work, no further attempt is made to register one of the two modalities to the other. Finally, the intensity of the extracted regions is rescaled linearly to the 0-255 range. The result of this region extraction stage is illustrated in Fig. 2.

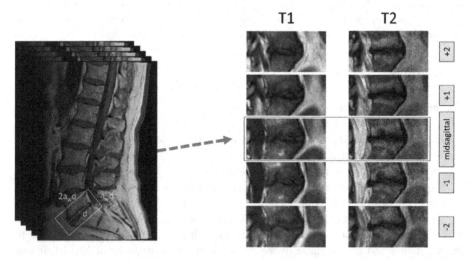

Fig. 2. Schematic illustration of the procedure for the extraction of the IVD volumes. The width of the IVD, its center and its orientation are given as input (left). Then, a region of aspect ratio 2:1 is extracted from five T1 and five T2 slices, symmetrically around the midsagittal slice (the two slices from the left side of the midsagittal, the midsagittal and the two slices from its right side). The result of this procedure is 10 aligned IVD regions, as shown on the right.

2.2   Network Architecture

A variant of VGG16 CNN of [15] is employed, with the following modifications to the vanilla architecture: (a) The size of the input layer is $112 \times 224 \times 6$; (b) A dropout layer is added after the last convolutional layer and (c) there is only one fully-connected layer before the softmax classification. The six channels of the input volume consist of three IVD regions extracted from the T1 slices and the corresponding three IVD regions from the T2 slices, in that order. An illustration of the employed architecture is presented in Fig. 3.

The weighted cross entropy is used as a loss function in all the conducted experiments. Due to the imbalanced representation of the classes in the dataset, the contribution of every training sample to the loss function is weighted according to its class. These class weights are set to be inversely proportional to the frequency of the respective class in the training set.

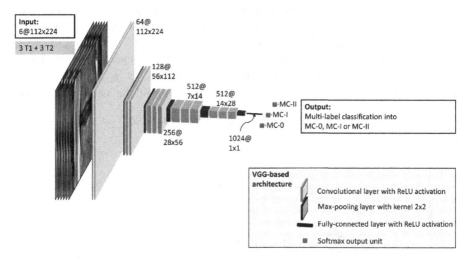

Fig. 3. Schematic illustration of the VGG16 architecture of [15] as employed in the single-stage variant of the present work. The input to the CNN consists of six channels of size 112×224, populated with the IVD regions that are extracted from the three T1 and and three T2 slices. The output is a softmax layer of three units, corresponding to the grades MC-0, MC-I, MC-II. Each layer of the architecture is represented with a rectangle, whose width is proportional to the number of feature maps in the layer. For the two-stage variant, the CNN architectures of the first and the second stage differ only on the final classification layer (two output units instead of three).

2.3   Mixup

An important challenge in this study is the lack of a satisfactory number of cases with a non-background label. Only 123 IVD regions (22.3% of the total number) in our dataset have a label which is not MC-0, with 84 of them labeled as MC-II. We attempt to partially address this problem by using the so-called *mixup* strategy, introduced in [16].

The mixup approach was motivated in [16] by the desire to reduce the oscillating predictive behavior of a trained classification model when it encounters samples that fall outside of its training set. The basic idea is the following: Given two training samples $S_1 = (x_1, y_1)$ and $S_2 = (x_1, y_2)$ where $y_1, y_2 \epsilon [0, 1]^M$ are 1-hot vectors and M is the number of classes in the problem, a new training sample S_m is formed by a linear interpolation of S_1, S_2:

$$S_m = (x_m, y_m) = (\lambda \cdot x_1 + (1 - \lambda) \cdot x_2, \lambda \cdot y_1 + (1 - \lambda) \cdot y_2), \lambda \in [0, 1] \qquad (1)$$

Or more concisely:

$$S_m = \lambda \cdot S_1 + (1 - \lambda) \cdot S_2, \lambda \in [0, 1] \qquad (2)$$

Where the weight λ is a random variable. When λ is very close to either 0 or 1, S_m will very similar to one of the original training samples, whereas values near 0.5 lead to maximum blending. Following [16], λ is drawn from a beta distribution, giving flexibility on specifying how aggressively new mixup samples are formed. An illustration of the mixup procedure is shown in Fig. 4.

Although after the application of mixup the target y_m is no longer an 1-hot vector, it can still be treated as a probabilistic distribution. Indeed, let $y_1 = [y_{1,1}, \cdots y_{1,M}]$, $y_2 = [y_{2,1}, \cdots y_{2,M}]$, $y_m = [y_{m,1}, \cdots y_{m,M}]$ be the elements of the target vectors we interested in. The original targets y_1 and y_2 are 1-hot vectors, so $\sum_{i=1}^{M} y_{1,i} = \sum_{i=1}^{M} y_{2,i} = 1$. Then:

$$\sum_{i=1}^{M} y_{m,i} = \sum_{i=1}^{M} \lambda \cdot y_{1,i} + (1 - \lambda) \cdot y_{2,i}$$

$$= \lambda \cdot \sum_{i=1}^{M} y_{1,i} + (1 - \lambda) \cdot \sum_{i=1}^{M} y_{2,i} = \lambda + (1 - \lambda) = 1$$

Also, the elements $y_{m,i}$ are all positive since $\lambda, (1 - \lambda) > 0$. Therefore, the target y_m can be treated as a discrete probability distribution over the M classes. This is important because it allows us to continue using the cross-entropy as a loss function for training the network, which is the standard choice for classification tasks.

In practice, mixup can be understood as a data augmentation method [16] and it can be implemented with minimal modifications to the standard training pipeline. In particular, for every training mini-batch, a random permutation of it is constructed and the λ values are sampled from the beta distribution. Then, the original mini-batch and its permuted version are multiplied with λ and $(1 - \lambda)$ and they are added together to form the mixup mini-batch.

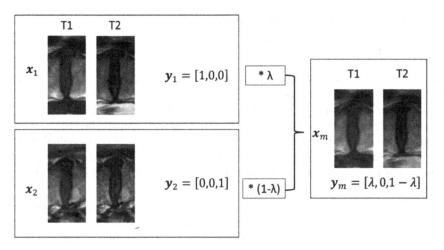

Fig. 4. Illustration of the generation of the mixup training samples for a 3-class classification scenario (MC-0, MC-I, MC-II). On the left, two training samples from the original mini-batch with labels MC-0 and MC-II (top to bottom). The two training samples are linearly interpolated with weights λ and $(1 - \lambda)$ to form a mixup training sample. In this example, $\lambda = 0.769$. The entire IVD volumes are interpolated (for convenience, only one pair of T1 and T2 slices are shown on the figure).

2.4   IVD Level Grading

A straightforward approach for predicting the label of a certain IVD level would be to pass the isolated T1 and T2 IVD volumes (of five slices each) to the network and use the prediction of the network as the prediction for the MC of that level. In practice however, we found out that the accuracy is improved if narrower volumes are used as input. The adopted strategy is as follows: firstly, from the original T1 and T2 IVD volumes of five slices, three sub-volumes are constructed with three consecutive IVD regions each. The constructed T1 and T2 sub-volumes are combined, forming three volumes of size $112 \times 224 \times 6$. Then, these three combined volumes are passed in succession to the network in order to get one prediction for each of them. If all of these predictions are MC-0, the assigned grade for this particular IVD level is MC-0. Otherwise, it is the grade that corresponds to the most confident prediction.

Such an approach can be justified on the grounds that it mimics the process that a human rater is following when rating a given pair of T1 and T2 sequences: One examines one T1 slice and one T2 slice at a time, in order to assess whether MC intensity patterns are present or not. The two adjacent slices are also taken into account in order to decide whether any pinpointed pattern is consistent with the presence of a MC or it is an unrelated artifact. If it is decided that a MC is present, this is enough to assign a MC grade to whole IVD level, even if the detected pattern is not visible throughout the sagittal length of the endplate.

3   Experimental Design and Results

3.1   Dataset

The dataset of this study consists of a fully anonymized dataset of 92 pairs of T1 and T2 sequences. These sequences were acquired using a variety of protocols, including fat-suppressed T1 and T2, some of them employing the Dixon method. The inclusion criteria were the following: (a) The entire sacrolumbar region should be visible; (b) any deformities of the spinal curvature should be limited enough for a midsagittal slice to still be definable and (c) no implants should be present on the lumbar region of the spine. All of these sequences were sagittally acquired, with the total number of slices per sequence being in the 9–17 range.

The endplate regions of six spinal levels from T12/L1 to S1/L5 of every case were rated from two spine surgeons according to the MC grading system with every case being rated by exactly one rater. The acquisition of the ground truth was guided by the following criteria:

(a) Only the five slices closest to the midsagittal one were taken into consideration during grading;
(b) Only intensity changes of the bone marrow that extend from an endplate were graded as a MC;
(c) The MC pattern must be visible in at least two adjacent sagittal slices for an endplate region to be graded as MC-I or MC-II.

Similar criteria have been used in literature in order to standardize the annotation process [4, 8, 10]. The localization of the IVDs that is required for the extraction of the IVD regions was performed with the help of a manual, approximate segmentation of the IVDs. The orientation of each IVD was given by the first component of a principal component analysis (PCA) on the corresponding binary segmentation mask of the IVD and the IVD center by the centroid of the mask.

3.2   Evaluation

The dataset was split in 9 folds; 8 folds have the sequences of 10 patients and one fold of 12 patients. A standard 9-fold cross-validation study was then conducted and the achieved accuracy was compared with the annotations provided by the experts. Therefore, every case participated exactly once in the study as a member of a testing fold, permitting the computation of the evaluation metrics on the whole dataset.

The principal evaluation metric that was used is the *average-per-class accuracy* (APCA), which is especially suited for unbalanced classification tasks. In particular, let $ACC_{MC-0}, ACC_{MC-I}, ACC_{MC-II}$ by the achieved accuracies for the classes MC-0, MC-I and MC-II respectively. Then, the APCA will be:

$$ACC_{APC} = \frac{ACC_{MC-0} + ACC_{MC-I} + ACC_{MC-II}}{3} \tag{3}$$

We also record the accuracy of detecting whether certain degree of MC is present, i.e. the accuracy on the union of the MC-I and MC-II classes. We will denote this measurement with ACC_{MC}. The APCA for this binary classification task is:

$$ACC_{APC,bin} = \frac{ACC_{MC-0} + ACC_{MC}}{2} \tag{4}$$

Finally, the total, unweighted accuracy ACC is also reported, i.e. the rate of the correct automatic classifications.

3.3   Multiclass Classification vs. Two-Stage Classification

In addition to the classification pipeline as presented in the previous section, we evaluated an alternative scheme where the multiclass CNN classifier is replaced by two binary classifiers, assembled in a two-stage classification fashion. In particular, the first-stage binary classifier makes a prediction on whether the given IVD volume has a MC grade of MC-0 or not. If the first-stage classifier does not detect a MC-0 grade, the second-stage classifier further classifies the same IVD volume into MC-I or MC-II. Except for the final softmax layer, both of these binary classifier share exactly the same architecture as the multiclass classifier, including the size of the input IVD volume. Both pipelines were evaluated with and without the application of mixup strategy.

3.4   Hyperparameters

The values of the hyperparameters were set using two splits of a subset of 78 cases of the dataset into 70 training and 8 testing cases. The width of the extracted IVD regions was set to be 1.7 times the width of the IVD. The parameter alpha of the beta distribution of mixup was set to 0.1 for all experiments. Mixup was applied indiscriminately to all the MC classes, thus all the combinations of MC classes were possible during the creation of the mixup mini-batch. The dropout rate was set to 0.2. The mini-batch for the training of the multiclass classifier and of the first-stage classifier was formed from the IVD volumes of three cases of the training set. The size of the mini-batch of the second-stage classifier was set to six IVD volumes, drawn from all the IVD volumes of the training set with a non-MC-0 label. The weights of all the network were initialized from a VGG16 network pre-trained on ImageNet [17]. The networks were trained for 40 epochs when mixup strategy was not used and for 80 epochs when mixup strategy was used. The difference in the number of epochs was due to our observation that, when mixup is applied, more epochs are need for the training error to reach the same level (this observation agrees with [16]). When mixup was not used, the performance seemed to actually get worse when the network was trained to the same number of epochs (80), hence we decided to keep it much lower (40), in an attempt to make the comparison fair. Furthermore, as in [14], we noticed that the increased network capacity offered by the two additional fully-connected layers of the default VGG16 architecture hurt the performance, therefore we kept only one fully-connected layer before the softmax layer.

Similar to [14], extensive training-time data augmentation was applied: rotation of the IVD regions by ±7.5°, change of their scale by a factor of 0.8–1.2, displacement of their center by ±5 pixels in the coronal and axial dimensions, random flipping in the coronal direction with a probability of 0.5 and swapping of the order of the IVD regions in a volume with a probability of 0.5.

3.5   Results

Four variations of the proposed method were evaluated, corresponding to the four configuration combinations of using/not-using mixup and for multiclass/two-stage classification. The achieved evaluation scores are reported in Table 1. For the case of the two-stage classification, the ACC_{MC-0} and ACC_{MC} metrics depend only the performance of the first-stage classifier. On the other hand, the ACC_{MC-I} and ACC_{MC-II} metrics depend on both on the accuracy of the first-stage on detecting MCs and on the ability of the second-stage classifier to discriminate between MC-I and MC-II.

From this table, we can make some observations: firstly, the application of mixup resulted in an improvement in five out of the six recorded evaluation metrics, both in the multiclass and in the two-stage classification scheme. The metric that got worse in both scenarios was the accuracy on the MC-0 class (ACC_{MC0}). These results leave the impression that mixup improves the accuracy on the underrepresented classes, at the modest expense of the most common class.

The second observation is that the two-stage classification scheme seems to be performing better than the multiclass one. Even though ACC_{MC-II} got worse in the two-stage pipeline, leading to a worse ACC_{MC} too, the APCA is much higher (both the binary and the multiclass one), as well as the total accuracy.

Table 1. The achieved accuracies of the four variation of the pipeline (with and without mixup, multiclass vs. two-stage classification). All the shown values are percentages over the whole dataset. The number of IVD levels with labels MC-0, MC-I and MC-II is 429, 39, 84 respectively. The best values are highlighted with bold font.

	MC-0	MC-I	MC-II	MC-I + MC-II	APCA	APCA binary	Accuracy
Multiclass classifier							
No mixup	90.4	41.0	78.6	88.6	70.0	90.0	85.1
Mixup	88.8	59.0	**81.0**	**94.3**	76.2	91.6	85.5
Two-stage classification							
No mixup	**93.2**	51.3	71.2	87.8	71.6	90.5	86.8
Mixup	92.8	**64.1**	75.0	91.9	**77.3**	**92.3**	**88.0**

4   Discussion and Conclusion

This paper proposed a method for the automated detection of MC-I and MC-II in IVD regions. The four variants of the proposed method were evaluated in a standard 9-fold cross-validation setup with a heterogeneous dataset of 92 cases. The evaluation demonstrated the usefulness of the recently proposed mixup strategy for this type of classification task. Interestingly, a two-stage classification scheme achieved a generally better performance than a multiclass classification approach.

Despite the relatively small size of the dataset used, the proposed method seems to achieve a performance that is similar to or even better than those achieved by the state-of-the-art methods. In particular, the most performant variant achieved an accuracy of 88.0%, which compared favorably to the 87.8% accuracy of [12], the only other published method for the automatic MC multiclass grading. However, a direct comparison is difficult to make, since our dataset is different and smaller compared to the one used in [12] and we also opted to omit the MC-III grade from our study. On the other hand, when the proposed method is used as a binary detector for the presence or not of MCs, the achieved performance is very good, with an average-per-class accuracy of 92.3%, for the most performant variant.

Despite the success of the method in detecting the presence of MCs, their classification into MC-I or MC-II was proved to be a more challenging task for the present method: the average-per-class-accuracy of 77.3% leaves much to be desired. The accuracy on the MC-I class was particularly low (64.1%), likely related to the small number of cases with such a grading on our dataset (39 in total).

As part of future work, we plan to collect and annotate additional cases, since we feel that this is a limiting factor of the current study. A larger dataset could hopefully allow us to consider MC-III in our study. Even though MC-III is clinically less significant, the etiology of MCs is still not well understood and an automated system for the identification of all the recognized MC types would be beneficial to MC-related research. From a technical standpoint, it would be also interesting to see if mixup remains effective on a larger dataset.

References

1. De Roos, A., et al.: MR imaging of marrow changes adjacent to end plates in degenerative lumbar disk disease. Am. J. Roentgenol. **149**(3), 531–534 (1987)
2. Modic, M.T., et al.: Degenerative disk disease: assessment of changes in vertebral body marrow with MR imaging. Radiology **166**(1), 193–199 (1988)
3. Modic, M.T., et al.: Imaging of degenerative disk disease. Radiology **168**(1), 177–186 (1988)
4. Wang, Y., Videman, T., Battié, M.C.: Modic changes: prevalence, distribution patterns, and association with age in white men. Spine J. **12**(5), 411–416 (2012)
5. Zhang, Y.-H., et al.: Modic changes: a systematic review of the literature. Eur. Spine J. **17**(10), 1289–1299 (2008)
6. Albert, H.B., et al.: Modic changes, possible causes and relation to low back pain. Med. Hypotheses **70**(2), 361–368 (2008)
7. Järvinen, J., et al.: Association between changes in lumbar Modic changes and low back symptoms over a two-year period. BMC Musculoskelet. Disord. **16**(1), 98 (2015)
8. Fayad, F., et al.: Reliability of a modified Modic classification of bone marrow changes in lumbar spine MRI. Jt. Bone Spine **76**(3), 286–289 (2009)
9. Crockett, M.T., et al.: Modic type 1 vertebral endplate changes: injury, inflammation, or infection? Am. J. Roentgenol. **209**(1), 167–170 (2017)

10. Wang, Y., et al.: Quantitative measures of Modic changes in lumbar spine magnetic resonance imaging: intra-and inter-rater reliability. Spine **36**(15), 1236–1243 (2011)
11. Vivas, E.L.A., et al.: Application of a semiautomatic classifier for Modic and disk hernia changes in magnetic resonance. Coluna/Columna **14**(1), 18–22 (2015)
12. Jamaludin, A., Kadir, T., Zisserman, A.: Automatic Modic changes classification in spinal MRI. In: Vrtovec, T., Yao, J., Glocker, B., Klinder, T., Frangi, A., Zheng, G., Li, S. (eds.) CSI 2015. LNCS, vol. 9402, pp. 14–26. Springer, Cham (2016). https://doi.org/10.1007/978-3-319-41827-8_2
13. Jensen, T.S., Sorensen, J.S., Kjaer, P.: Intra-and interobserver reproducibility of vertebral endplate signal (Modic) changes in the lumbar spine: the Nordic Modic consensus group classification. Acta Radiol. **48**(7), 748–754 (2007)
14. Jamaludin, A., Kadir, T., Zisserman, A.: SpineNet: automatically pinpointing classification evidence in spinal MRIs. In: Ourselin, S., Joskowicz, L., Sabuncu, Mert R., Unal, G., Wells, W. (eds.) MICCAI 2016. LNCS, vol. 9901, pp. 166–175. Springer, Cham (2016). https://doi.org/10.1007/978-3-319-46723-8_20
15. Simonyan, K., Zisserman, A.: Very deep convolutional networks for large-scale image recognition. arXiv preprint arXiv:1409.1556 (2014)
16. Zhang, H., et al.: mixup: beyond empirical risk minimization. arXiv preprint arXiv:1710.09412 (2017)
17. Deng, J., et al.: ImageNet: a large-scale hierarchical image database. In: IEEE Conference on Computer Vision and Pattern Recognition, CVPR 2009. IEEE (2009)

Error Estimation for Appearance Model Segmentation of Musculoskeletal Structures Using Multiple, Independent Sub-models

Paul A. Bromiley[1]([✉]), Eleni P. Kariki[2], and Timothy F. Cootes[1]

[1] Centre for Imaging Sciences, School of Health Sciences, University of Manchester, Manchester, UK
{paul.bromiley,timothy.f.cootes}@manchester.ac.uk
[2] Radiology and Manchester Academic Health Science Centre, Manchester University Hospitals NHS Foundation Trust, Manchester, UK
eleni.kariki@mft.nhs.uk

Abstract. Segmentation of structures in clinical images is a precursor to computer-aided detection (CAD) for many musculoskeletal pathologies. Accurate CAD systems could considerably improve the efficiency and objectivity of radiological practice by providing clinicians with image-based biomarkers calculated with minimal human input. However, such systems rarely achieve human-level performance, so extensive manual checking may be required. Their practical utility could therefore be increased by accurate error estimation, focusing manual input on the images or structures where it is needed. Standard techniques such as the minimum variance bound can estimate random errors, but provide no way to estimate any systematic errors due to model fitting failure.

We describe the use of multiple, independent sub-models to estimate both systematic and random errors. The approach is evaluated on vertebral body segmentation in lateral spinal images, demonstrating large (up to 50%) and significant improvements in the accuracy of error classification with concurrent improvements in annotation accuracy. Whilst further work is required to elucidate the definition of "independence" in this context, we conclude that the approach provides a valuable component for appearance model based CAD systems.

1 Introduction

Standard statistical techniques exist to estimate errors on model fitting processes. For example, in maximum likelihood or equivalent techniques such as cross-correlation, the covariance matrix of the fitted model parameters is bounded by (e.g. [2])

$$C_{\theta_{r,s}}^{-1} \leq - < \frac{\partial^2 \log L}{\partial \theta_r \partial \theta_s} > = - \frac{\partial^2 \log L}{\partial \theta_r \partial \theta_s} \bigg|_{\theta=\theta_{max}} \tag{1}$$

© Springer Nature Switzerland AG 2019
G. Zheng et al. (Eds.): CSI 2018, LNCS 11397, pp. 53–65, 2019.
https://doi.org/10.1007/978-3-030-13736-6_5

where L is the likelihood function, r, s index a vector of parameters θ, and the equality on the right-hand side is true in the large N limit. This is known as the Minimum Variance Bound (MVB) and has been successfully applied to estimate errors on registration, patch-matching and landmark localisation algorithms (e.g. [5,9,15]). However, Eq. 1 shows that the covariance matrix on the fitted model parameters is bounded by the width of the log-likelihood function about the fitted optimum. It is not sensitive to any systematic error introduced by unmodeled modes of variation in the data, or fit failure due to convergence on a local optimum, as shown in Fig. 1. In general, without either a prior distribution on the systematic errors or a perfect model, there is no way to estimate systematic errors since they cannot be randomly sampled.

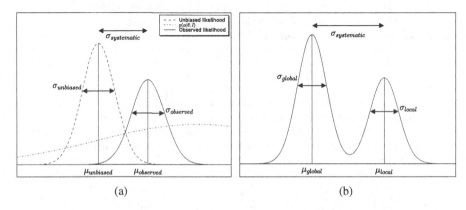

(a)   (b)

Fig. 1. (a) Unmodeled modes of variation in the data introduce a biasing parameter α and so a prior term $p(\alpha|\theta, I)$ where I is the query image and θ the model parameters. (b) Use of a local, rather than global, optimiser may allow fitting to converge on a local optimum. In either case, the minimum variance bound estimates the accuracy with which a given optimum has been found, which is dependent on the width of that optimum (σ_{biased} or σ_{local}) about its mean (μ_{biased} or μ_{local}), but is not sensitive to the systematic error $\sigma_{systematic}$.

It is often the case in medical image analysis that the most significant errors are systematic, and induced by the use of imperfect models that cannot account for all of the non-noise variation in the data. Such models can be considered as existing on sub-spaces in the space of the perfect model i.e. they span some, but not all, of the modes of variation of that model, and each has a systematic error on a given query image as a result. However, if multiple models could be produced, independent in the sense that they exist on different sub-spaces, their results would include random samples from the population of all possible systematic errors. The standard techniques for random error analysis could then be applied to estimate the systematic errors. This approach has been successfully applied to landmark annotation for Computed Tomography (CT) images using patch-based rigid registration [6]. Here, we explore its application to appearance model segmentation of musculoskeletal images.

As an exemplar task, Random Forest Regression Voting Constrained Local Models (RFRV-CLMs) [13] were applied to segment vertebrae in Dual-Energy X-ray Absorptiometry (DXA) spinal images, to support classification of osteoporotic vertebral fractures (VFs). This combination of method and application had several advantages. Osteoporosis is a common, degenerative disease that increases the risk of fragility fractures, which most frequently occur in the vertebrae, wrists and hips. Approximately 40% of postmenopausal Caucasian women are affected, increasing their lifetime fragility fracture risk to as much as 40% [14]. The impact of the disease is expected to grow as the population ages [7]. Early identification of osteoporotic VFs is therefore clinically important. However, the false negative rate for VF identification is high. A recent audit at a large UK hospital revealed a reporting rate of 36% on CT images [12], and similarly low rates have been reported elsewhere [1]. VF identification on CT images may be opportunistic. However, a recent multi-centre, multinational prospective study on VF reporting for lateral radiographs found a false negative rate of 34% [8]. The potential utility of computer-aided diagnostic (CAD) systems for VF identification in clinical images is therefore high. RFRV-CLMs have previously been applied to this task in both DXA [3] and CT [4] demonstrating state-of-the art annotation and classification accuracy. However, these publications showed that model fitting failure limited classification accuracy. A reliable method to identify such errors would considerably improve the practical utility of VF CAD systems based on RFRV-CLMs, avoiding much of the need for manual inspection and/or correction of the results.

2 Method

Random Forest Regression Voting Constrained Local Models. In the interests of brevity we provide only a summary of the RFRV-CLM and refer the reader to [13] for full details. RFRV-CLMs match a series of landmark points, described by a statistical shape model (SSM), to a query image. They consist of a SSM and a set of independent, local models of the image intensities around each point. The latter are aligned to the query image independently, with the SSM providing a global constraint. The training data consists of a set of images, each annotated with n homogeneous points x_l, where $l = 1...n$. The sets of points are first aligned to remove non-shape variation using e.g. a similarity transformation. The shape in each aligned image is represented as a vector comprising the concatenated coordinates of the points in that image. Principal Component Analysis (PCA) is applied to these vectors to extract the main modes of variation $\mathbf{P}$. A linear model is then constructed giving x_l as the mean point position $\bar{x}_l$ in a suitable reference frame, plus some proportion b of each of the modes of variation

$$\mathbf{x}_l = T_\theta(\bar{\mathbf{x}}_l + \mathbf{P}_l \mathbf{b} + \mathbf{r}_l) \tag{2}$$

where $\mathbf{P}_l$ is the sub-matrix of $\mathbf{P}$ relevant to l, and $\mathbf{b}$ are referred to as the shape parameters. T_θ is the transformation, with parameters θ, from the reference frame to the query image, and $\mathbf{r}_l$ allows small deviations from the model. Fitting to a query image $\mathbf{I}$ proceeds by optimising a quality of fit Q over parameters $\mathbf{p} = \{\mathbf{b}, \theta, \mathbf{r}_l\}$, where

$$Q(\mathbf{p}) = \Sigma_{l=1}^{n} C_l(T_\theta(\bar{\mathbf{x}}_l + \mathbf{P}_l\mathbf{b} + \mathbf{r}_l)) \quad \text{s.t.} \quad \mathbf{b}^T\mathbf{S}_b^{-1}\mathbf{b} \leq M_t \quad \text{and} \quad |\mathbf{r}_l| < r_l \quad (3)$$

The threshold M_t is a shape constraint and is applied to the Mahalanobis distance of $\mathbf{b}$, using the covariance matrix $\mathbf{S}_b$ of the $\mathbf{b}$ from the training data, and r_l is a threshold on the residuals. The cost images C_l are produced by Random Forest (RF) regression voting. For each l, patches are sampled from the image at a set of random displacements from $\mathbf{x}_l$ in the reference frame, Haar-like features are derived from the patches, and a RF regressor is trained to predict the displacement from the features. During fitting each RF is scanned across the image around the current estimate of the point location and the predicted displacements are entered into a voting array C_l.

Data Collection and Manual Annotation. The dataset used in the evaluation consisted of 320 DXA VF assessment (VFA) images scanned on various Hologic (Bedford MA) scanners, with manual annotation of 33 landmarks on each vertebra from T7 to L4; see Fig. 2 for example images. Each vertebra was also classified by an expert radiologist into one of five groups (normal, deformed but not fractured, and grade 1 (mild), 2 (moderate), and 3 (severe) fractures as defined by Genant et al. [10].

RFRV-CLM Training and Fitting. The training procedures and parameters described in [3] were used. RFRV-CLMs were trained to model landmarks on triplets of neighbouring vertebrae, using training data from all levels between T7 and L4 such that the models could fit any level. Two-stage, coarse-to-fine models were used with two trees in the first stage and 15 in the second. Fitting to query images was initialised using manual annotations of vertebral body centroids. The shape constraint in Eq. 3 was removed in the last iteration of second-stage fitting to avoid correlated errors between the landmarks. The model was fitted to all triplets of centroids between T7 and L4, and landmarks from the central vertebrae of each (plus the extremal vertebrae on the first and last triplets) were concatenated to produce a segmentation of the vertebrae.

Error Estimation Methodology. The evaluation of the proposed approach to systematic error detection was based on comparing two model-training regimes. The first, referred to below as "multi-model", evaluated error estimators based on multiple, independent models. Weak independence was induced by training models on independent data sets; see Sect. 4 for comments on potential routes to formally inducing strong independence. The data set was divided into eighths and models were trained on each. Therefore, seven models trained on independent sets of images were available to fit each query image, producing seven independent estimates $\mathbf{x}_j$ for each landmark location. The final annotation was produced by taking the centroid $\mathbf{x}_c$ of the multiple estimates. An error estimator sensitive to any fit failures across the set of models was calculated as the root-mean-square (RMS) of the Euclidean distances between the individual estimates and their centroid, and is referred to below as RMS goodness-of-fit (RMSGOF)

$$\mathbf{x}_c = \frac{1}{k}\sum_{j=0}^{k}\mathbf{x}_j \qquad RMSGOF = \sqrt{\frac{1}{k}\sum_{j=0}^{k}(\mathbf{x}_j - \mathbf{x}_c)^2} \qquad (4)$$

For comparison, a standard four-fold cross validation was also performed and is referred to below as "single model". Here, models were trained on 3/4 of the data and tested on the remaining 1/4, such that one model was tested on each query image. Since RFRV-CLMs contain regressors capable of predicting the location of the landmark given patches of image data, a simple goodness-of-fit measure sensitive only to random errors was produced by applying the regressor at the optimised point position to estimate the residual; this is referred to below as RGOF (residual GOF). RGOF was also calculated for the multi-model approach by taking the mean of the RGOF from each of the multiple model fits for a given point, and a combined GOF, or CGOF, was produced by taking the product of the mean RGOF and the RMSGOF.

In both cases, the true error on the RFRV-CLM annotations was calculated as the Euclidean distance to the corresponding manual annotation. This is referred to below as point-to-point, or P2P, error. The RF parameters were kept consistent between the single model and multi-model approaches. In addition, multi-model training used all vertebral triplets from each training image whilst single-model training used only one; since T7 to L4 annotation provided eight triplets per image, this ensured that the number of training samples used for each model was consistent across both approaches.

Vertebral Fracture Classification. VF classification was performed using a simple approach based on six-point morphometry [11]. The anterior H_a, middle H_m, and posterior H_p heights of each vertebral body were calculated as the Euclidean distances between the relevant landmark pairs. The predicted posterior body height $H_{p'}$ was also calculated from the posterior heights of the closest four annotated vertebrae by taking the largest of the four values, since fractures decrease vertebral height. Three ratios were then calculated to measure the relative height reductions at the anterior (wedge ratio, H_a/H_p), middle (biconcavity ratio, H_m/H_p) and posterior (crush ratio, $H_p/H_{p'}$) positions. The data were whitened by subtracting the median and dividing by the square root of the covariance matrix, estimated using the median absolute deviation. Normal vertebrae predominated, and so this was equivalent to whitening to the mean and standard deviation of the normal class, without using manual classifications. A simple classifier was then constructed by placing a threshold t_c on the Euclidean distance from the origin to separate the data into fractured and non-fractured classes, the latter including both normal and deformed vertebrae. Error estimates for classification were derived from RMSGOF, CGOF and RGOF by applying standard error propagation to the above calculation to produce a scaled estimate of the error HGOF on the length of the vector defined by the three whitened height ratios R_w, R_b and R_c, and calculating the ratio of this estimate to the distance of the data point from the decision boundary

$$ClassGOF = \frac{HGOF}{|t_c - \sqrt{R_w^2 + R_b^2 + R_c^2}|} \tag{5}$$

3 Evaluation

Figure 2 shows example images and serves as a flow diagram illustrating the method. Taking the original images (a, f) as input, together with manual annotations of vertebral body centres, RFRV-CLMs are fitted to produce high-resolution annotations of the vertebral bodies as a precursor to VF classification.

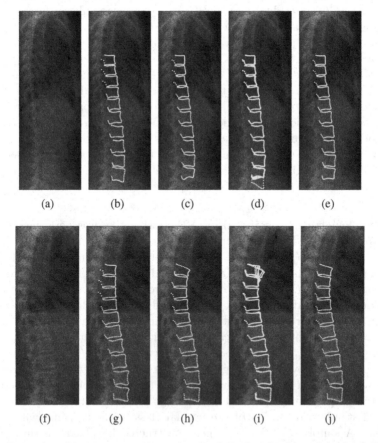

(a)   (b)   (c)   (d)   (e)

(f)   (g)   (h)   (i)   (j)

Fig. 2. Examples of image annotation using single and multiple models. (a, f) Original images. (b, g) Manual annotations of T7 to L4. (c, h) Automatic annotation using a single RFRV-CLM. (d, i) Automatic annotations from multiple, independent models. (e, j) Centroids of the multiple estimates for each landmark.

Comparing manual annotations (b, g) to automatic annotations produced by a single model (c, h), it can be seen that some vertebra (L4 in (c) and T7 in (h)) are poorly fitted, leading to the appearance of reduction in anterior vertebral body height that leads to misclassification of these normal vertebrae as fractured. Since these errors are systematic, rather than random, techniques based on the MVB will not identify them. However, if multiple, independent sub-models are fitted (d, i), they can serve to sample the systematic errors. The centroids of the multiple estimates for each point (e, j) serve as the final annotation.

The first stage of the evaluation focused on estimating the mean P2P error across each vertebral body. Figure 3 shows scatterplots of the mean single-model RGOF and multi-model RMSGOF for each vertebra against the vertebral mean P2P error. The correlation coefficient was 0.54 for the vertebral mean single model RGOF, 0.50 for the mean multi-model RGOF, 0.63 for the mean RMS-GOF, and 0.67 for the mean CGOF, indicating that the RMSGOF is more strongly correlated to the P2P error than the RGOF. The CGOF resulted in a small improvement in correlation, indicating that there is some independent information between the RGOF and RMSGOF.

To provide a more quantitative interpretation of the various error estimators, they were used to construct binary classifiers. The ground truth classification for each vertebra was produced by imposing a threshold on mean P2P error, set to the 95th percentile of the error distribution, corresponding to 2.2 mm. Figure 4 shows ROC curves produced by applying a threshold to the error estimators and comparing the classification to the ground truth. Error estimators based on multiple models resulted in a large and significant increase in classification accuracy, e.g. raising the precision at 50% recall from 42.1% for a single-model RGOF to 59.3% for RMSGOF and 63.8% for CGOF.

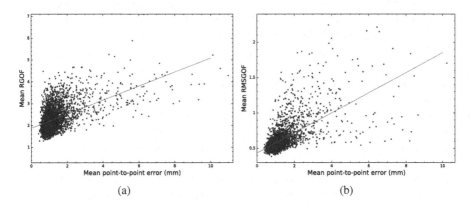

(a)   (b)

Fig. 3. Goodness-of-fit (GOF) measures vs. the P2P errors on automatically annotated points: (a) mean single-model RGOF; (b) RMSGOF. Each graph also shows a linear fit to the data.

The results discussed so far indicate that the use multiple, independent sub-models is helpful in error estimation. However, the effect on the accuracy of

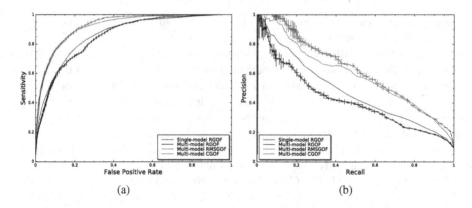

Fig. 4. ROC curves for binary classifiers of mean vertebral error using various error estimators. The ground truth was provided by a threshold on the mean vertebral P2P error corresponding to the 95th percentile of its distribution.

point localisation must also be evaluated. Since each of the multiple sub-models is trained on a smaller set of images, it might be expected that the resultant regressors would provide point location estimates with larger errors. In practice, the opposite was found. Figure 5 shows CDFs of the mean vertebral P2P errors divided by vertebral classification, for both single and multiple models. In general, multi-model annotation proved to be slightly more accurate than single model annotation, although the differences were small. This also accounts for the difference in accuracy between single and multi-model RGOF in Fig. 4; the multi-model annotation makes fewer errors and so they are more difficult to identify. However, Fig. 6 shows ROC curves for a six-point morphometry classifier applied to both the manual annotations and automated annotations from single and multi-models. Multi-model VF classification was significantly more accurate, approximately halving the difference compared to classification from manual annotations.

To investigate this difference more thoroughly, several additional model training strategies were applied, and the results are also shown in Fig. 6. As described in Sect. 2, in the experiments described up to this point single models were trained on one vertebral triplet from each of the training images whilst, when training multiple models, the training images were divided into eighths and one model was trained on each, using all of the vertebral triplets. Furthermore, the dimensions of the RFs were consistent, with two trees in the first stage and fifteen in the second stage. Therefore, the number of trees and training samples for each individual model was consistent but, as an ensemble, the multiple sub-models had seven times more trees and training samples available. To test whether this accounted for the difference in accuracy between the single and multi-model approaches, additional single models were trained with all vertebral triplets from all images, and with increased numbers of trees in the first and second stages, and the results are shown in Fig. 6. Increasing the training

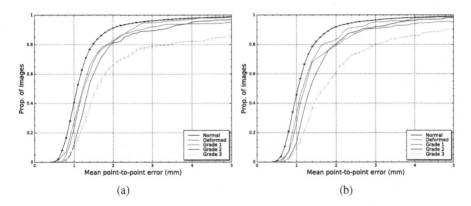

Fig. 5. Cumulative distribution functions of the vertebral mean P2P error on RFRV-CLM annotations using a single model (a) and multiple models (b), for each vertebral classification.

sample approximately halved the difference between the single and multi-model approaches, and increasing the number of trees in each stage produced further but smaller increases in accuracy. However, the single model still failed to achieve the accuracy of the multi-model approach. Conversely, the size of the model on disk increased dramatically. For example, the first stages of the multi-models were on average 290 MB; single-model first stages were 230 MB for two trees and one triplet per image and, when using all triplets, 1.2 GB for 2 trees and 5.0 GB for 8 trees, making the latter impractically large. This indicates that dividing training samples between multiple, independent models provides a more efficient way in which to use large data sets. The single models used in the remaining experiments reverted to the training strategy described in Sect. 2.

The final stage of the evaluation focused on identifying errors in the 6-point morphometry fracture classification. Classification and error estimation were performed as described in Sect. 2. A classification threshold t_c (an operating point in Fig. 6) giving 90% sensitivity was selected. A second threshold was applied to the ClassGOF (derived from CGOF) to classify the VF classification as accurate or erroneous. The ground truth was provided by the manual classification of each vertebra, and the threshold on ClassGOF was varied to produce the ROC curves shown in Fig. 7(a).

Comparison of the results from single and multi-model error estimation for VF classification is complicated by the fact that, as shown in Fig. 6, multi-model fracture classification is more accurate, and so the number of errors to be detected is smaller. However, in contrast to the results for classifying errors on vertebral mean errors, the multi-model approach did not provide significantly more accurate error estimation for VF classification compared to the single-model approach. To illustrate why this occurred, Fig. 8 shows the distributions of multi-model annotation error, across all vertebrae and images, for each of the 33 landmarks. However, instead of P2P error, the figure shows the

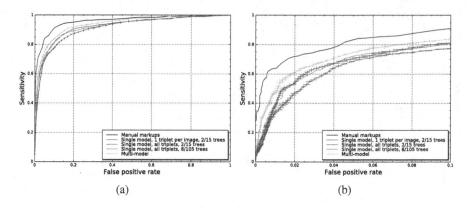

(a)   (b)

Fig. 6. ROC curves of osteoporotic VF classification using 6-point morphometry, for both manual landmarks and various automated annotations; (b) shows a detail from (a).

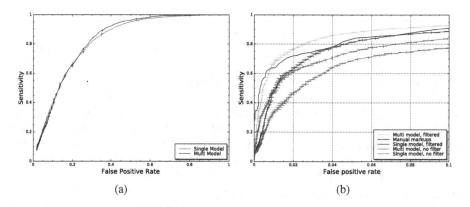

(a)   (b)

Fig. 7. (a) ROC curves showing the accuracy of error classification on the results of VF classification using 6-point morphometry. (b) ROC curves of osteoporotic VF classification using 6-point morphometry, for both manual landmarks, the single and multi-model automatic annotations, and these automatic annotations after filtering out results detected as erroneous by an error classifier.

point-to-curve (P2C) errors i.e. the minimum Euclidean distance between each point and a piecewise-linear curve through the manual annotations. Large P2C errors, where the points move away from the vertebral body edge, are predominantly found on the anterior side and the pedicle, whilst the points used in VF classification are more accurate, implying they are less subject to fit failure. Therefore, mean vertebral P2P error estimation benefits from the use of RMSGOF and the sensitivity of the technique to systematic error/fit failure, whilst error estimation for VF classification does not. However, the multi-model approach did not result in significantly worse error estimation.

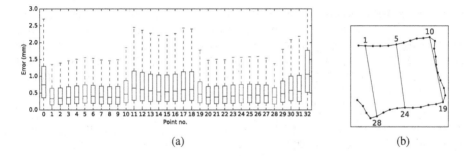

(a)   (b)

Fig. 8. (a) Box-and-whisker plots of the point-to-curve errors on the multi-model centroid estimates of each point. The points shown in red are those used to estimate heights for fracture classification, as shown in (b). (Color figure online)

To provide a more quantitative interpretation of the use of single and multi-model error estimation for VF classification, Fig. 7(b) shows ROC curves of the 6-point morphometry fracture classifier applied to the manual, single and multi-model annotations, and to the single and multi-model annotations after removal of all vertebrae that were classified as inaccurate by the error classifier. This reflects the use of the error estimation as a component of a CAD system, identifying potentially inaccurate classifications for manual checking and correction. The threshold used for error classification was set to the operating point that gave 10% false positive rate in Fig. 7(a). When combined with error classification, single-model fracture classification was more accurate than multi-model classification without error classification, and multi-model fracture classification was more accurate than classification based on manual annotations. At an operating point of 90% sensitivity in the filtered, multi-model ROC curve, fewer than 20% of the vertebrae were labeled for manual inspection and only 5.65% of the fractured vertebrae were misclassified both as normal and accurate i.e. 94.35% of fractured vertebrae were either correctly classified or identified as inaccurate.

4   Conclusion

The use of shape and appearance models to segment structures in clinical images is well established and has been proposed as the basis for clinical decision support systems for a number of musculoskeletal pathologies. However, these systems rarely achieve human-level accuracy. Reliable estimates of the errors on the results would significantly increase their practical utility by highlighting the images or structures requiring human input. However, this requires error estimation techniques sensitive not only to random errors but also to systematic errors such as model fitting failures.

This work has demonstrated the use of multiple, independent sub-models as a route to estimation of systematic errors on appearance model fitting. The underlying approach is not novel but we believe that this is the first time it has been applied to appearance models. Using vertebral body segmentation and osteoporotic VF classification in DXA images as an example, the approach was shown to be as accurate as an RF regressor in estimating random errors, but significantly more accurate in estimating systematic errors. The use of multiple sub-models also resulted in improvements in annotation accuracy by allowing more efficient use of large training sets. The combination of these effects allowed multi-model VF classification based on 6-point morphometry with error filtering to exceed the accuracy of classification from manual annotations whilst rejecting fewer than 20% of the vertebral segmentations, implying that it could have practical utility in appearance model based CAD systems.

The work described here acts as a proof-of-concept but is preliminary. For example, we have not explored the variations in annotation and error estimation accuracy with varying numbers of sub-models. More significantly, the definition of independence of the sub-models was not explored. Some degree of independence was ensured by using independent training sets for each model. However, a true definition of independence would require that each model existed on a separate sub-space of the shape and appearance space. Independence might therefore be maximized by permuting the assignment of training samples to models to maximize the distances between the sub-spaces as measured using the Grassmanian. In the case of spinal images, constraints would be required to ensure this did not separate training samples by vertebral level and produce sub-models that could not fit the whole spine. We intend to explore this in future work.

Acknowledgments. This publication presents independent research supported by the NIHR Invention for Innovation (i4i) programme (grant no. II-LB_0216-20009). The views expressed are those of the authors and not necessarily those of the NHS, the NIHR or the Department of Health and Social Care. The authors acknowledge the invaluable assistance of Mrs Chrissie Alsop, Mr Stephen Capener, Mrs Imelda Hodgkinson, Mr Michael Machin, and Mrs Sue Roberts, who performed the manual annotations.

References

1. Adams, J.E.: Opportunistic identification of vertebral fractures. J. Clin. Densitom. **19**(1), 54–62 (2016)
2. Barlow, R.: Statistics: A Guide to the Use of Statistical Methods in the Physical Sciences. Wiley, Hoboken (1989)
3. Bromiley, P.A., Adams, J.E., Cootes, T.F.: Localisation of vertebrae on DXA images using constrained local models with random forest regression voting. In: Yao, J., Glocker, B., Klinder, T., Li, S. (eds.) Recent Advances in Computational Methods and Clinical Applications for Spine Imaging. LNCVB, vol. 20, pp. 159–171. Springer, Heidelberg (2015). https://doi.org/10.1007/978-3-319-14148-0_14
4. Bromiley, P.A., Kariki, E.P., Adams, J.E., Cootes, T.F.: Fully automatic localisation of vertebrae in CT images using random forest regression voting. In: Yao, J., Vrtovec, T., Zheng, G., Frangi, A., Glocker, B., Li, S. (eds.) CSI 2016. LNCS, vol. 10182, pp. 51–63. Springer, Cham (2016). https://doi.org/10.1007/978-3-319-55050-3_5

5. Bromiley, P.A., Pokric, M., Thacker, N.A.: Empirical evaluation of covariance estimates for mutual information coregistration. In: Barillot, C., Haynor, D.R., Hellier, P. (eds.) MICCAI 2004. LNCS, vol. 3216, pp. 607–614. Springer, Heidelberg (2004). https://doi.org/10.1007/978-3-540-30135-6_74
6. Bromiley, P.A., Schunke, A.C., Ragheb, H., Thacker, N.A., Tautz, D.: Semi-automatic landmark point annotation for geometric morphometrics. Front. Zool. **11**(61), 1–21 (2014)
7. Burge, R., Dawson-Hughes, B., Solomon, D.H., Wong, J.B., King, A., Tosteson, A.: Incidence and economic burden of osteoporosis-related fractures in the United States 2005–2025. J. Bone Miner. Res. **22**, 465–475 (2007)
8. Delmas, P.D., et al.: Underdiagnosis of vertebral fractures is a worldwide problem: the IMPACT study. J. Bone Miner. Res. **20**(4), 557–563 (2005)
9. Erdt, M., Steger, S., Wesarg, S.: Deformable registration of MR images using a hierarchical patch based approach with a normalized metric quality measure. In: 2012 9th IEEE International Symposium on Biomedical Imaging (ISBI), pp. 1347–1350 (2012)
10. Genant, H.K., Wu, C.Y., Kuijk, C.V., Nevitt, M.C.: Vertebral fracture assessment using a semi-quantitative technique. J. Bone Miner. Res. **8**(9), 1137–1148 (1993)
11. Jergas, M., Valentin, R.S.: Techniques for the assessment of vertebral dimensions in quantitative morphometry. In: Genant, H.K., Jergas, M., van Juijk, C. (eds.) Vertebral Fracture In Osteoporosis, pp. 163–188. University of California Osteoporosis Research Group, San Francisco (1995)
12. Kariki, E.P., Bromiley, P.A., Cootes, T.F., Adams, J.A.: Opportunistic identification of vertebral fractures on computed radiography: need for improvement. Osteoporos. Int. **27**(S2), 621 (2016)
13. Lindner, C., Bromiley, P.A., Ionita, M., Cootes, T.F.: Robust and accurate shape model matching using random forest regression-voting. IEEE TPAMI **37**(9), 1862–1874 (2015)
14. Rachner, T.D., Khosla, S., Hofbauer, L.C.: Osteoporosis: now and the future. Lancet **377**(9773), 1276–1287 (2011)
15. Söhn, M., et al.: Model-independent, multimodality deformable image registration by local matching of anatomical features and minimization of elastic energy. Med. Phys. **35**(3), 866–878 (2008)

Automated Segmentation of Intervertebral Disc Using Fully Dilated Separable Deep Neural Networks

Huan Wang, Ran Gu, and Zhongyu Li[✉]

School of Mechanical and Electrical Engineering,
University of Electronic Science and Technology of China, Chengdu, China
zhongyu.emerald@gmail.com

Abstract. Accurate segmentation of intervertebral discs is a critical task in clinical diagnosis and treatment. Despite recent progress in applying deep learning to the segmentation of multiple natural image scenarios, addressing of the intervertebral disc segmentation with a small-sized training set are still challenging problems. In this paper, a new framework with fully dilated separable convolution (FDS-CNN) is proposed for the automated segmentation of the intervertebral disc using a small-sized training set. Firstly, a fully dilated separable convolutional network is designed to effectively prevent the loss of context information by reducing the number of down-sampling. Secondly, a multi-modality data fusion and augmentation strategy are proposed, which can increase the number of samples, as well as make full use of multi-modality image data. Experimental results validate the proposed framework in the MICCAI 2018 Challenge on Automatic Intervertebral Disc Localization and Segmentation from 3D Multi-modality MR Images, demonstrating excellent performance in comparison with other related segmentation methods.

Keywords: Intervertebral disc · Dilated separable convolution · Semantic segmentation · Multi-modality data fusion

1 Introduction

Disc degeneration is likely to cause various back problems, where accurate segmentation of intervertebral discs (IVDs) from MR images is a critical task in clinical diagnosis and treatment [1]. Recent advances of deep learning techniques have greatly facilitated the segmentation of MR images. Given a MR image (either 2D or 3D), deep learning systems can automatically localize and segment all related lesions end-to-end without user intervention. However, for the segmentation of intervertebral discs, the large range of IVD shapes and the limited

---

H. Wang and R. Gu—Equal contribution.

© Springer Nature Switzerland AG 2019
G. Zheng et al. (Eds.): CSI 2018, LNCS 11397, pp. 66–76, 2019.
https://doi.org/10.1007/978-3-030-13736-6_6

number of available datasets pose significant challenges in practical applications, e.g., MICCAI 2018 Challenge on Automatic Intervertebral Disc Localization and Segmentation. Especially, for this challenge, the IVD shapes are dramatically different even in the same type of IVDs, where the availably small-sized dataset (only includes 64 3D MR images) are hard to support the training of deep segmentation model. Therefore, new methods need to be developed to address the above challenges for the IVD segmentation.

Early studies on IVD segmentation [2–4] have been done by manually extracted features, where these hand-crafted features are dependent on expert knowledge that can be subjective and unreliable. Recently, with the development of deep learning, many effective methods have been proposed in the field of image segmentation. Lin et al. proposed RefineNet [5], which explicitly exploits all the information available along the down-sampling process to enable high-resolution prediction using long-range residual connections. Zhao et al. [6] proposed PSPNet, which uses the pyramid pooling module to obtain multi-scale features. Wang et al. [7] proposed HDC to reduce the gridding issue caused by the standard dilated convolution operation with a simple and effective method. In particular, Deeplabv3 and Deeplabv3+ proposed by Chen et al. [8,9] achieved a better performance on the PASCAL VOC 2012 semantic image segmentation dataset by using spatial pyramid pooling and dilated convolution.

Unlike natural images, medical images usually lack sufficient annotations to differentiate images or pixels from multi-modality imaging devices [20]. In practice, it is difficult to collect a large number of annotated samples to train the segmentation model. Because of the problem, the above methods have difficulty in adapting to medical images. Recently, researchers have proposed multiple methods focused on the medical image segmentation. For example, Chen et al. [10] proposed a 3D full convolutional network (FCN) for IVD localization and segmentation. Li et al. [11] proposed a multi-scale and modality dropout-learning framework to segment IVDs from four modality MR images. Zeng et al. [12] proposed a deeply supervised multi-scale fully convolutional network, which uses a multi-scale deeply supervised method to automatically segment and locate IVDs and using transfer learning to improve the performance of the deep model. Liao et al. [13] proposed a multi-task 3D FCN combined with a bidirectional recurrent neural network to automatically segment vertebrae from the CT images. In addition, Zeng et al. [14] proposed a deeply supervised 3D fully convolutional network to segment the proximal femur in 3D MR images. However, the problem of losing a lot of contextual information is still well unsolved due to the excessive use of down-sampling. Meanwhile, with the number of network layers increases, the parameters will also increase dramatically, which can increase the computational complexity of the whole network.

Taking the above problems into account, this paper proposes a new framework with fully dilated separable convolution (FDS-CNN) for the automatic segmentation of IVDs, using small-sized training set from multi-modality MR images. Firstly, we design a fully dilated separable convolution network that replaces all standard convolutions with dilated separable convolution, and prevents the loss of contextual information by reducing the number of down-sampling. At the same time, in the case of ensuring the segmentation performance, the network parameters can be effectively reduced. Subsequently, to make full use of the characteristics of multi-modality data, we propose a multi-modality data fusion and augmentation strategy, which can increase the number of samples in a simple and effective manner, improving the generalization performance of the network. Finally, by drawing on the idea of the attention model [15], we use pre-processing networks to pre-segment the spine and make the network more focused on the places of interest.

This paper is organized as follows. In Sect. 2, we present the proposed framework in detail. Then, our framework is evaluated using the MICCAI 2018 IVD Segmentation Challenge Data Set in Sect. 3. Finally, Sect. 4 draws the conclusion and discusses future works.

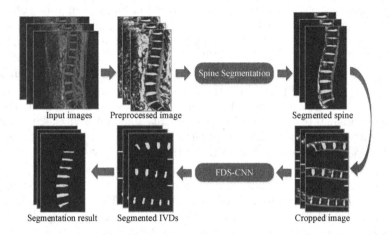

Fig. 1. Overview of the fully automated intervertebral disc segmentation framework.

2   Methodology

Figure 1 presents the overall framework for the automated IVDs segmentation. In order to suppress the complex background interference of multi-modality data, the framework mainly includes two parts, i.e., (1) segmenting the spine out of the original images; (2) segmenting the IVDs using the FDS-CNN. Besides, we propose a multi-modality data fusion and augmentation strategy which can make full use of the characteristics of multi-modality data to effectively increase the number of training samples. Accordingly, in this section, we first present the method for spine segmentation, and then introduce our proposed FDS-CNN structure in detail. Finally, we introduce the multi-modality data fusion and augmentation strategy.

2.1   U-Net for Spine Segmentation

According to Fig. 1, we notice that the original IVD MR image has complicated backgrounds, which may influence the performance of our segmentation model. In order to make the IVD segmentation more focused on the area of interest, we first introduce a pre-processing network to segment the spine from the original image. The network is based on U-net [16] with BN [17] layers after each convolution to speed up network convergence. U-net is a simple and effective semantic segmentation network. It extracts high-level semantic information from images through step-by-step down-sampling, and then restores the size of the image, predicting the results step-by-step through up-sampling and skip connection. Through the pre-processing network, spine images with the area of interests can be obtained. Accordingly, before the segmentation of IVDs, pre-segmentation of spine regions mainly has two advantages, i.e., (1) the subsequent FDS-CNN only need to tackle the area of interest; (2) the computational complexity can be greatly reduced. This idea is similar to the widely used attention model [15] in the field of natural language processing. The model puts more attention on the area of interest to obtain more details of the target and ignore other useless information.

2.2   Convolutional Network with Fully Dilated Separable Convolution

After the pre-segmentation of spine regions, we use the FDS-CNN for the accurate segmentation of IVDs. The FDS-CNN first employs an improved Xception [18] as the encoder network to extract high-level semantic information, extracting multi-scale features based on a spatial pyramid model. Then, it can recover the lost context information using a skip connection. Compared to previous works [6,8,9], the propose framework has multiple improvements in the corresponding modules to adapt the IVD segmentation task with only small-sized training set. In particular, our network replaces all convolutions with dilated separable convolutions, which can greatly reduce the number of parameters of the network and effectively extend the field of receptivity. Moreover, our network does not need any pre-training, which can still achieve superior performance with small-sized training set. The following of this section will introduce the implementation details of our network.

Dilated Separable Convolution. The main idea of dilated convolution is to insert "holes" (zeros) between pixels to enlarge the field of convolutional kernels, which enable dense feature extraction in deep CNNs [7]. Dilated convolution allows us to explicitly control the resolution at which feature responses are computed within deep convolutional neural networks [8]. It can effectively expand the field of view in each filter without increasing parameters and computational complexity. We can obtain enough receptive fields through dilated convolution without down-sampling. Therefore, the loss of context information due to down-sampling can be well avoided. Besides, depthwise separable convolution separates the standard convolution into depthwise convolution followed by a

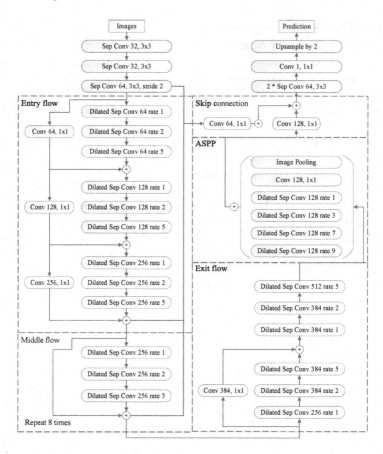

Fig. 2. The structure of the convolutional network with fully dilated separable convolution (FDS-CNN), including modified Xception, ASPP, skip connection, etc.

pointwise convolution. Specifically, the depthwise convolution performs a spatial convolution independently for each input channel, while the pointwise convolution is employed to combine the output from the depthwise convolution [9]. This decomposition can greatly reduce the computational complexity of the model. In our designed FDS-CNN architecture, we use 3×3 depthwise separable convolutions, which can not only have less computation complexity (i.e., 8 to 9 times less) than the standard convolution, but also maintain similar performance as the standard convolution [19]. Our dilated separable convolution combines the depthwise separable convolution and the dilated convolution. The dilated separable convolution embeds the characteristics and inherits the advantages of these two kinds of convolutions. For example, the dilated separable convolution can be treated as a dilated convolution, effectively increasing the receptive field of the network, which also has fewer parameters in comparison with the standard convolution.

Modified Xception. The Xception model [18] has achieved excellent performance in image classification and segmentation tasks. Recently, Chen et al. [9] applied the modified Xception model to address the semantic segmentation and achieve excellent performance. In our solution, we continue to make further three changes to the Xception model and apply it to address the IVD segmentation task. First, we replace all convolutions in the Xception model with dilated separable convolutions and use only one down-sampling in the entire model. Second, in order to further improve the computation efficiency, we reduce the number of all feature maps by half. Third, in order to effectively expanding the receptive field, the dilated separable convolutions in each layer are assigned with different rates. The modified Xception is shown in Fig. 2.

Additionally, we adopt other two strategies to further improve the performance of FDS-CNN, i.e., Atrous Spatial Pyramid Pooling (ASPP) [6,9] and Skip Connection. As shown in Fig. 2, we replace all convolutions in the spatial pyramid structure with dilated separable convolutions, where the rate of dilated separable convolutions in each layer can be modified accordingly. Subsequently, the 1×1 convolutions are applied to three low-level features, which are the output of the third layer convolution, the output of the enter flow and the output of the middle flow, respectively. Then they are concatenation with high-level features. After the concatenation, we apply two 3×3 separable convolutions and one 1×1 convolution to refine the features followed by a simple bilinear upsampling with the factor of 2.

2.3 Multi-modality Data Fusion and Augmentation

For the small-sized training set, the segmentation model is easy to over-fitting. For this problem, a general solution is to increase the number of samples by rotating each image, thereby improving the generalization performance of the model. Although this method can well increase the number of samples, it cannot use the characteristics of multi-modality data itself. Therefore, we develop a new method for multi-modality data fusion and augmentation. According to Fig. 3, from (a–b), it can be seen that multi-modality images have different modalities for the same object (IVD). However, the shape and position of objects inside the image have not changed. Therefore, it is possible to use the feature of multi-modality data to construct new modality. From (e–h), by simply adding the corresponding pixel values from the original two modality images, images with new modality can be obtained. This strategy can not only increase the number of samples, but also fuse different modalities to better represent IVDs. We will verify the performance of the multi-modality data fusion and augmentation strategy in the experimental part.

3   Experiments

3.1   Experimental Setting

We evaluated the proposed framework on the dataset from MICCAI 2018 Challenge of Automatic Intervertebral Disc Localization and Segmentation [21]. The

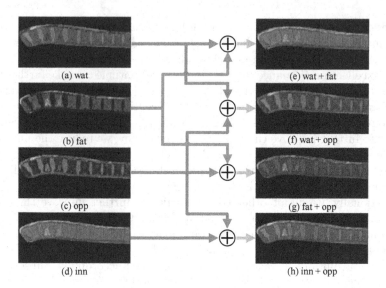

Fig. 3. Schematic diagram of multi-modality data fusion and augmentation strategy.

data set contains 3D images from 8 patients scanned using a 1.5-Tesla MRI scanner at two different times. In addition, each 3D multi-modality MRI data set contains four aligned high-resolution 3D volumes: in-phase (inn), opposed-phase (opp), fat and water (wat) images. There are in total 64 high-resolution 3D MRI volume data. For each IVD, ground truth labels are provided in the form of binary mask with pixel level annotation.

For the data pre-processing , the multi-modality fusion and augmentation strategy discussed above is used to create a variety of sample data, which can significantly increase the number of training samples. Meanwhile, traditional data augmentation strategies such as image rotation are also employed. In order to improve the performance of the model when dealing with blurred imaging samples, we randomly selects images before the image input network, i.e., randomly selecting 0%–15% of pixels of the image, assigning random-sized values. With the increasing training batches, each image has different levels of noise, which can increase the diversity of the sample. Besides, each image is normalized using min-max normalization.

For the spine segmentation, in order to reduce the influence of complex backgrounds, we employ a pre-segmentation network to extract spine regions from original images. Spine segmentation network adopt U-net model [16] that has widely applied in image segmentation. After the spine segmentation, we cut the image into 112×128 sub-maps to train the deep neural network. Additionally, the FDS-CNN outputs the predicted image of the same size (112×128) as the training data, where this paper uses the splicing method to restore the predicted image to its original size. In the training of FDS-CNN, we employ the open source architecture from Keras, using the Adam optimization function, where the learning rate are set as 1E-4, with the batch_size of 16. Our deep neural networks are implemented using Keras on a Linux system with two Nvidia 1080Ti GPUs.

3.2 Evaluation

This paper uses cross-validation to evaluate the performance of the framework. Due to the multi-modality images are scanned at different times, most images from same patients are similar which cannot be set as training and testing data respectively. Therefore, for the cross-validation, the training and testing data will not include the multi-modality images of the same patient. The data set contains in total 16 image data from 8 patients. For each round of validation, 12 image data from 6 patients are selected for training, and the remaining 4 image data are used for testing. In this paper, four groups of cross-validation are performed in each experiment, and dice overlap coefficients are used to evaluate the prediction results of the framework. In the following, we first evaluate the effectiveness of the proposed FDS-CNN, and then verify the performance of the multi-modality data fusion and augmentation strategy.

Table 1. Performance comparison of our network and two benchmarks on the IVD segmentation dataset under different modalities.

	Wat	Fat	Inn	Opp	Mean
Deeplabv3+ [9]	0.8309	0.8124	0.8257	0.8243	0.8235
U-net [16]	0.9107	0.8651	0.9051	0.8992	0.8953
FDS-CNN	**0.9111**	**0.8853**	**0.9055**	**0.9062**	**0.9021**

Effectiveness of FDS-CNN. To validate the effectiveness of the proposed FDS-CNN, we compare our approach with 2 benchmark methods: U-net [16] and Deeplabv3+ [9]. For these two benchmarks, as the scanned MRIs are single-channel grayscale images, the input dimensions of networks are modified accordingly. Meanwhile, we reduce the number of channels in the convolutional layers, adding the BatchNormal layer to accelerate the convergence of U-net. All three networks using the same training and augmentation strategies. Table 1 records the dice score of three comparative methods. According to Table 1, the proposed FDS-CNN achieves a mean dice overlap coefficient (MDOC) of 90.21%, where the U-net and Deeplabv3+ only achieve MDOC of 89.53% and 82.35%, respectively. The results demonstrate that the proposed FDS-CNN can achieve better performance in the IVD segmentation task with small-sized training set. Meanwhile, we notice that the accuracy of segmentation achieved by Deeplabv3+ is obviously less than that of U-net. This indicates that Deeplabv3+, which performs well in natural image segmentation tasks, can not well adapt the small-sized medical image data sets. Figure 4 illustrates a randomly selected example with corresponding segmentation results using the proposed FDS-CNN. According to Fig. 4, our network can achieve the segmentation for IVDs with reasonable results. It is worth pointing out that the accuracy of fat modality in these networks is lower than that of other modalities. This is because the IVDs in the fat modality have low resolution, which can reduces the accuracy of segmentation.

Table 2. The performance of the fused modalities on the trained model.

Wat+Opp	Fat+Opp	Wat+Inn	Inn+Opp	Mean
0.9122	0.9086	0.9121	0.9140	0.9117

Table 3. Results without multi-modality data fusion and augmentation.

Wat	Fat	Inn	Opp	Mean
0.9096	0.8818	0.8984	0.8975	0.8973

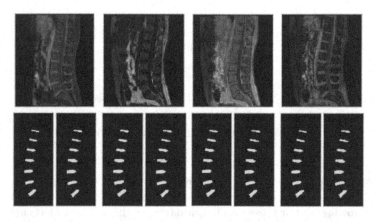

Fig. 4. Examples of segmentation results from the validation data set. From left to right, they are wat, fat, inn, and opp modalities. The second row is their segmentation results (left) and the corresponding ground truth (right).

Validation of Multi-modality Data Fusion and Augmentation. We adopt two protocols to validate the effectiveness of the proposed multi-modality data fusion and augmentation strategy. We first use the new modality to test the segmentation accuracy in the model, and then testing the performance of the model without using multi-modality data fusion and augmentation strategy. According to Table 2, the fused new modalities achieves the MDOC of 91.17%, which is better than the original results, i.e., 90.21% as shown in Table 1. Moreover, the segmentation accuracy of each new modality is also higher than the original modality. In particular, the fat+opp modality is 2.33% higher than the fat modality result, which can be treated as a preferable solution for the problem of low resolution of the fat modality. This validates that the proposed multi-modality data fusion and augmentation strategy can effectively fuse different features from multiple modalities to improve the accuracy of segmentation. As illustrated in Table 3, the model only achieves MDOC of 89.73% when the multi-modality data fusion and augmentation strategy was not used. Moreover, the segmentation accuracy of each modality is also lower than the results in Table 1. This shows that the multi-modality data fusion and augmentation strategy can provide rich multi-modality data for the network to support the learning of dis-criminant information, thereby improving the segmentation results of IVDs.

4   Conclusion

In this paper, a new framework with fully dilated separable convolution (FDS-CNN) is proposed for the IVD multi-modality image segmentation with small-sized training set. Compared with other segmentation networks, the proposed FDS-CNN can achieve superior performance in small-sized training set without pre-training. By investigating the information from multi-modality image data, this paper proposes a novel solution for the multi-modality image augmentation, i.e., multi-modality data fusion and augmentation strategy, which can increase the number of samples and improve the performance of the segmentation model. Experiments on MICCAI 2018 IVD Localization and Segmentation Challenge demonstrate the effectiveness and superiority of the proposed framework, in comparison with other state-of-the-arts.

References

1. Luoma, K., Riihimäki, H., Luukkonen, R., Raininko, R., Viikarijuntura, E., Lam-minen, A.: Low back pain in relation to lumbar disc degeneration. Spine **25**(4), 487–492 (2000)
2. Ben Ayed, I., Punithakumar, K., Garvin, G., Romano, W., Li, S.: Graph cuts with invariant object-interaction priors: application to intervertebral disc segmen-tation. In: Székely, G., Hahn, H.K. (eds.) IPMI 2011. LNCS, vol. 6801, pp. 221–232. Springer, Heidelberg (2011). https://doi.org/10.1007/978-3-642-22092-0_19
3. Law, M.W., Tay, K., Leung, A., Garvin, G.J., Li, S.: Intervertebral disc segmenta-tion in MR images using anisotropic oriented flux. Med. Image Anal. **17**(1), 43–61 (2013)
4. Chevrefils, C., Chériet, F., Grimard, G., Aubin, C.-E.: Watershed segmentation of intervertebral disk and spinal canal from MRI images. In: Kamel, M., Campilho, A. (eds.) ICIAR 2007. LNCS, vol. 4633, pp. 1017–1027. Springer, Heidelberg (2007). https://doi.org/10.1007/978-3-540-74260-9_90
5. Lin, G., Milan, A., Shen, C., Reid, I.: RefineNet: multi-path refinement networks for high-resolution semantic segmentation. In: IEEE Conference on Computer Vision and Pattern Recognition (CVPR), pp. 5168–5177 (2017)
6. Zhao, H., Shi, J., Qi, X., Wang, X., Jia, J.: Pyramid scene parsing network. In: CVPR, pp. 2881–2890 (2017)

7. Wang, P., et al.: Understanding convolution for semantic segmentation. arXiv preprint, arXiv: 1702.08502 (2017)
8. Chen, L.C., Papandreou, G., Schroff, F., Adam, H.: Rethinking Atrous convolution for semantic image segmentation. arXiv preprint, arXiv: 1706.05587 (2017)
9. Chen, L.C., Zhu, Y., Papandreou, G., Schroff, F., Adam, H.: Encoder-decoder with Atrous separable convolution for semantic image segmentation. arXiv preprint, arXiv: 1802.02611. (2018)
10. Chen, H., Dou, Q., Wang, X., Qin, J., Cheng, J.C.Y., Heng, P.A.: 3D fully convolutional networks for intervertebral disc localization and segmentation. In: MICCAI Workshop MIAR, pp. 375–382 (2016)
11. Li, X., Dou, Q., Chen, H., Fu, C.W., Heng, P.A.: Multi-scale and modality dropout learning for intervertebral disc localization and segmentation. In: MICCAI Workshop CSI, pp. 85–91 (2016)
12. Zeng, G., Zheng, G.: DSMS-FCN: a deeply supervised multi-scale fully convolutional network for automatic segmentation of intervertebral disc in 3D MR images. In: Glocker, B., Yao, J., Vrtovec, T., Frangi, A., Zheng, G. (eds.) MSKI 2017. LNCS, vol. 10734, pp. 148–159. Springer, Cham (2018). https://doi.org/10.1007/978-3-319-74113-0_13
13. Liao, H., Mesfin, A., Luo, J.: Joint vertebrae identification and localization in spinal CT images by combining short-and long-range contextual Information. IEEE Trans. Med. Imaging **37**(5), 1266–1275 (2018)
14. Zeng, G., Yang, X., Li, J., Yu, L., Heng, P.-A., Zheng, G.: 3D U-net with multi-level deep supervision: fully automatic segmentation of proximal femur in 3D MR images. In: Wang, Q., Shi, Y., Suk, H.-I., Suzuki, K. (eds.) MLMI 2017. LNCS, vol. 10541, pp. 274–282. Springer, Cham (2017). https://doi.org/10.1007/978-3-319-67389-9_32
15. Bahdanau, D., Cho, K., Bengio, Y.: Neural machine translation by jointly learning to align and translate. arXiv preprint arXiv:1409.0473 (2014)
16. Ronneberger, O., Fischer, P., Brox, T.: U-Net: convolutional networks for biomedical image segmentation. In: Navab, N., Hornegger, J., Wells, W.M., Frangi, A.F. (eds.) MICCAI 2015. LNCS, vol. 9351, pp. 234–241. Springer, Cham (2015). https://doi.org/10.1007/978-3-319-24574-4_28
17. Ioffe, S., Szegedy, C.: Batch normalization: accelerating deep network training by reducing internal covariate shift. In: ICML, pp. 448–456 (2015)
18. Chollet, F.: Xception: Deep learning with depthwise separable convolutions. arXiv preprint, arXiv: 1610.02357 (2017)
19. Howard, A.G., Zhu, M., Chen, B., Kalenichenko, D., Wang, W., Weyand, T., et al.: Mobilenets: efficient convolutional neural networks for mobile vision applications. arXiv preprint, arXiv: 1704.04861 (2017)
20. Li, Z., Zhang, X., Müller, H., Zhang, S.: Large-scale retrieval for medical image analytics: a comprehensive review. Med. Image Anal. **43**, 66–84 (2018)
21. IVDM3Seg Homepage. https://ivdm3seg.weebly.com

Intensity Standardization of Skeleton in Follow-Up Whole-Body MRI

Jakub Ceranka[1,2(✉)], Sabrina Verga[1,3], Frédéric Lecouvet[4], Thierry Metens[5], Johan de Mey[6], and Jef Vandemeulebroucke[1,2]

[1] Department of Electronics and Informatics (ETRO),
Vrije Universiteit Brussel (VUB), Plainlaan 2, 1050 Brussels, Belgium
jceranka@etrovub.be
[2] imec, Kapeldreef 75, 3001 Leuven, Belgium
[3] Department of Electronics, Information and Bioengineering, Politecnico di Milano, Milan, Italy
[4] Institut de Recherche Experimentale et Clinique (IREC),
Université catholique de Louvain, Louvain-la-Neuve, Belgium
[5] Department of Radiology, ULB-Hôpital Erasme,
Université Libre de Bruxelles (ULB), Brussels, Belgium
[6] Department of Radiology, Universitair Ziekenhuis Brussel, Brussels, Belgium

Abstract. The value of whole-body MRI is constantly growing and is currently employed in several bone pathologies including diagnosis and prognosis of multiple myeloma, musculoskeletal imaging and evaluation of treatment response assessment in bone metastases. Intra-patient follow-up MR images acquired over time do not only suffer from spatial misalignments caused by change in patient positioning and body composition, but also intensity inhomogeneities, making the absolute MR intensity values inherently non-comparable. The non-quantitative nature of whole-body MRI makes it difficult to derive reproducible measurement and limits the use of treatment response maps. In this work, we have investigated and compared the performance of several standardization algorithms for skeletal tissue in anatomical and diffusion-weighted whole-body MRI. The investigated method consists of two steps. First, the follow-up whole-body image is spatially registered to a baseline image using B-spline deformable registration. Secondly, an intensity standardization algorithm based on a histogram matching is applied to the follow-up image. Additionally, the use of a skeleton mask was introduced, in order to focus the accuracy of algorithms on a tissue of interest. A linear piecewise matching method using masked skeletal region showed a superior performance in comparison to the other evaluated intensity standardization methods. The proposed work helps to overcome the non-quantitative nature of whole-body MRI images, allowing for extraction of important image parameters, visualization of whole-body MR treatment response maps and assessment of severity of bone pathology based on MR intensity profile.

Keywords: Whole-body MRI · Intensity standardization · Skeletal imaging

© Springer Nature Switzerland AG 2019
G. Zheng et al. (Eds.): CSI 2018, LNCS 11397, pp. 77–89, 2019.
https://doi.org/10.1007/978-3-030-13736-6_7

1   Introduction

The value of whole-body magnetic resonance imaging (MRI) in skeletal imaging is constantly growing and is currently getting more interest in investigation of several bone pathologies, including diagnosis and prognosis of multiple myeloma [1], bone marrow in paediatric age [3], musculoskeletal imaging [6] and evaluation of treatment response assessment in bone metastases [2,8,11].

Due to its high resolution, whole-body coverage and high sensitivity MRI can provide excellent definition of anatomical structures and underlying skeletal pathologies. Additionally, in combination with a follow-up scan, it allows for monitoring of changes in patients body composition and disease involvement providing reliable treatment response assessment parameters (i.e. change in cancer volume, number of metastases) and image response maps.

Follow-up MR images acquired in the same scanner do not only suffer from spatial misalignments caused by different patient positioning and changes in patients' body composition over time, but also intensity inhomogeneities, making the absolute MR intensity values inherently non-comparable. Therefore, due to the non-quantitative nature of MRI, intensities cannot be compared from one acquisition to another making it impossible to derive reproducible intensity measurements containing interpretable information. Standardized images can not be displayed with fixed windows without the need of per-case adjustment. Additionally, they limit the use of treatment response maps only to quantitative MR modalities, such as MR apparent diffusion coefficient (ADC) calculated using diffusion-weighted images. In order to successfully compare a baseline and a follow-up whole-body scan, both limiting factors have to be overcome, usually via the means of image post-processing techniques.

Whereas, intra-patient whole-body spatial image misalignment can be compensated by image registration [6,17], inter-scan intensity inhomogeneities bring a challenging problem. In the literature, few authors have described different intensity standardization methods for MR images, however most of the work was done in the field of neuroimaging, limiting the application perspective to a very specific domain and much smaller field of view.

Nyúl et al. [10] proposed a linear piecewise method of matching image histograms of brain images. First, a number of intensity landmarks representing statistical points (percentiles, modes) are found in the reference and target image histogram. Secondly, both image landmarks are mapped on the common reference intensity space using a piecewise linear transform.

Robitaille et al. [14] proposed a method similar to Nuyl with a different landmark detection algorithm. The method incorporates tissue spatial intensity information derived from the segmentation image allowing for detection of more precise, tissue specific landmarks.

Jäger et al. [5] represented a group of multi-modal reference and target brain images as an n-D joint probability histogram. The next step involved deformable registration of obtained n-D histograms, which provided the deformation field matrix. The latter was used to standardize intensity inhomogeneities between the reference and target image stack. Additionally, a method was adapted for whole-body MRI images.

In this work, we propose an extension of existing intensity standardization methods maximizing the intensity similarity of skeletal structures in whole-body MRI together with an extensive quantitative evaluation. A strong validation criterion of mean absolute difference is introduced, allowing for direct quantification of intensity profile separation. The performance of the proposed algorithm was compared with the state-of-the-art methods.

2   Materials and Methods

The skeleton standardization methodology consist of two steps. First, the follow-up whole-body image is spatially registered to a baseline image. Accurate alignment of baseline and follow-up images improves the similarity of the intensity histograms limiting the influence of intra-scan anatomical differences. Additionally, it allows for the introduction of strong validation criteria based on voxelwise intensity comparison, such as the mean absolute intensity difference. Secondly, four different image intensity standardization methods were implemented and validated, aiming for equalization of skeleton intensity profiles.

2.1   Spatial Registration

In order to spatially align the baseline and the follow-up whole-body image and compensate for the aforementioned spatial misalignment, image registration was used.

Registration was performed in a pairwise manner, taking the baseline whole-body image as the reference image, f, and a follow-up image as a moving image, g. The aim was to solve an optimization problem finding a spatial transformation $\mathcal{T}$ over the parameters μ, according to the following equation:

$$\hat{\mu} = \arg \min_{\mu} \mathcal{C}_{x \in \Omega} \Big(f(x), g(\mathcal{T}_\mu(x)) \Big) . \tag{1}$$

In (1), the spatial coordinate x is taken from the overlapping region Ω, in which we assumed an intensity interpolation scheme for the discrete images f and g. The registration is guided by the minimization of the chosen cost function $\mathcal{C}$. Due to non-quantitative nature of the MRI before intensity standardization, a mutual information (MI) cost function [9] was used:

$$\mathcal{D}_{MI}(f, g(\mathcal{T}_\mu)) = - \sum_{a,b} p_{fg}(a,b) \log \frac{p_{fg}(a,b)}{p_f(a)p_g(b)} , \tag{2}$$

where p_{fg} is the joint probability density function (PDF) of the images f and g, and p_f and p_g are the marginalised PDFs for the respective images. a and b are the image intensity values.

Three stage multi-resolution image registration consisting of a rigid, affine and deformable B-Spline [15] deformation was implemented in the freeware software package elastix [7]. For a deformable step, a bending energy penalty (BEP) was used [15]. Detailed registration parameters are provided in Table 1.

Table 1. Parameters used in the spatial registration step.

Parameter	Spatial registration		
Transform	Rigid	Affine	B-Spline
Metric	MI	MI	MI, BEP
Number of resolutions	3	4	4
Image pyramid schedule	4 2 1	8 4 2 1	8 4 2 1
B-Spline grid spacing	-	-	4 2 1 1
Final B-Spline grid spacing (mm)	-	-	15 15 15
Number of histogram bins	32	32	32
Metric 1 weight	1	1	1
Metric 2 weight	0	0	10
Max iterations	2000	2000	2000
Sampler	Random	Random	Random
Number of samples	2048	2048	2048

The registration was driven by high resolution 3D T_1 whole-body image and the resulting transformation field was used to map other modalities of lower image quality, i.e. diffusion-weighted images.

2.2 Intensity Standardization

We compared 5 different intensity standardization algorithms with increasing complexity based on histogram matching principle.

Method 1. Linear Scaling: Target image is linearly scaled to match the intensity distribution in a reference image. Because of the signal intensity outliers, we use the intensity range up the the 99.9% intensity percentile, which according to the Eq. 3 gives:

$$I_{LS} = I_{Rmin} \frac{I_T - I_{Tmin}}{I_{ToutlierPerc} - I_{Tmin}} (I_{RoutlierPerc} - I_{Rmin}). \tag{3}$$

Here, we denote I_R, I_T and I_{LS} as the reference, target and linearly scaled output image. I_{Rmin}, I_{Tmin}, $I_{RoutlierPerc}$ and $I_{ToutlierPerc}$ are the minimum intensity values and 99.9% intensity outlier percentile values of the reference and target image, respectively. Additionally, all other compared methods were initialized from the linearly scaled result in order to roughly align image intensity profiles before allowing for standardization with more degrees of freedom. Experiment was performed, showing a benefit of initialization by linear scaling.

Method 2. Piecewise Linear Matching of Intensity Histograms: The method is implemented similar to [10], where the basic idea is to find a linear piecewise mapping that deforms the follow-up image intensity histogram so that it matches a baseline image histogram using intensity landmarks. In the first step, five landmarks, L, representing intensity percentiles of the baseline and follow-up image are calculated. Here, a number of $n = 5$ evenly spaced percentile values was chosen, $L = [0, 20, 40, 60, 99.9]$. Second, a piecewise linear normalization is applied, mapping a follow-up image landmarks to corresponding baseline image landmarks, creating $n-1$ linear and independent transformations, each between two landmarks (see Fig. 1).

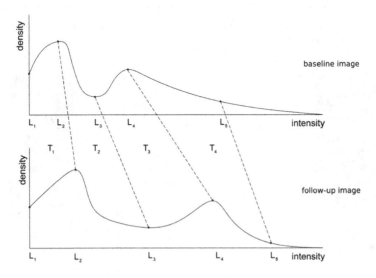

Fig. 1. Schematic representation of a linear piecewise transform. Two sets of landmarks L_{1-5} are detected in a reference and target image. Linear transformations T_{1-4} are used to standardize intensities between the images, mapping follow-up image intensities onto baseline image intensity profile.

Method 2.1. Piecewise Linear Matching of Masked Intensity Histograms: We propose a modification to the linear piecewise method by the introduction of the whole-body skeleton mask (see Sect. 2.3). Instead of taking all whole-body image voxels into account while calculating the intensity landmarks, only the masked tissues of interest will be used. Here, a 3D binary mask of the skeletal tissues is introduced, limiting excess of image information and focusing algorithm performance only on the chosen masked structure. Similar to method 2, five evenly spaced intensity percentiles were chosen as landmarks in the baseline and follow-up image, $L = [0, 20, 40, 60, 100]$, however, the range of intensities used was limited to the intensity range of the masked skeleton tissue. Later, as in method 2, piecewise normalization is performed taking into account updated landmark positions.

Method 3: Deformable Registration of Intensity Histograms: An image intensity histogram can be represented as a 1D image, where intensity values represent voxel count at each specific histogram bin. Therefore, the intensity standardization problem can be treated as a deformable image registration problem, aiming at finding a spatial transformation, $\mathcal{T}_\mu$, mapping a follow-up histogram image, $H(g)$, to a baseline intensity profile, $H(f)$, according to Eq. 1 (see Fig. 2). The resulting deformation field is used to correct intensities in the follow-up image [5]. Such method, gives more degrees of freedom compared to Method 2, allowing for smooth transformation and closer alignment of two intensity profiles. Here, a single-resolution deformable image registration with mean square difference cost function, bending energy penalty regularizer, histogram with 128 bins and a final B-Spline grid spacing of 30 pixels was used.

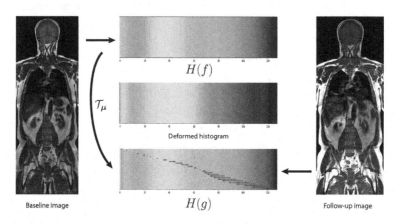

Fig. 2. Schematic representation of a deformable registration of two 1D histograms. The histogram of a follow-up image is deformably registered to the baseline image histogram. Obtained 1D deformation field (red arrows) is used to map intensities of the follow-up image onto baseline image intensity space. (Color figure online)

Method 3.1. Deformable Registration of Masked Intensity Histograms: The proposed method is a modification of method 3, where similarly to method 2.1, intensity histograms of the baseline and follow-up image are calculated only for the voxels included in the skeleton mask. Therefore, deformable registration is based only on intensities of interest, allowing for more precise intensity standardization transformation focusing on a chosen tissue of interest (i.e. bone).

2.3 Data Description

Experiments were performed on a 3D T_1 and diffusion-weighted whole-body images of prostate cancer patients with metastatic bone involvement and healthy volunteers. Each patient had one follow-up examination, with an approximate 3–9 months between consecutive scans. The follow-up images of healthy volunteers were acquired during the same day, in a separate scanning session. 5 whole-body image pairs (baseline + follow-up) of the same subject consisting of 4 image station covering roughly head, torso, pelvis and legs were acquired. Images were obtained as a routine examination performed in the Cliniques Universitaires Saint-Luc, Brussels and Universitair Ziekenhuis Brussel. The study was approved by the Institutional Ethics Board of both institutions.

MRI: Whole-body stations were composed after independent image station preprocessing, which involved noise filtering using anisotropic diffusion followed by bias field correction [18] both implemented as a standard **Insight Segmentation and Registration Toolkit** (ITK) filters. Additionally, interstation intensity standardization was applied by scaling the intensity distribution of neighbouring stations to 99.9% intensity percentile based on the common station overlay region prior to the composition of the whole-body image from separate stations.

Anatomical whole-body image station were acquired as a T_1 weighted spinecho sequence [12], with the following parameters: echo time (TE) = 8 ms, repetition time (TR) = 382 ms, matrix size of 480×480, pixel spacing 0.65 mm, slice thickness 1.19 mm. After the whole-body image reconstruction, spacing was equal to $1.2 \times 0.65 \times 0.65$ mm respectively in x, y and z direction with a matrix size of 210×1612–1705×768. Diffusion-weighted images were acquired with axial free breathing echo-planar DWI sequence (DWIBS) with a b-value equal to 1000 s/mm^2. Following sequence parameters were used: TR = 8421 ms, TE = 66 ms, slice thickness 6.1 mm, matrix size 192×192, pixel spacing 2.3 mm, FOV = 440×440 mm^2.

Skeleton Segmentation Mask: For each whole-body image pair (baseline and follow-up image), the skeleton segmentation for a reference image was delineated using first, the *'GrowCutEffect'* application from *Slicer* [4] followed by manual refinement. Additional smoothing was applied using morphological operations. Aiming at the specific applications for bone pathologies (metastatic bone disease, multiple melanoma), only a selected number of bones with high probability of involvement were considered. This involved clavicle, spine from C2 vertebra to sacrum, pelvis and both femur bones. Tubercular bone as well as the cortical bone were included. Figure 3 illustrates the anatomical reference of the bones that are considered in this study together with corresponding manual segmentations.

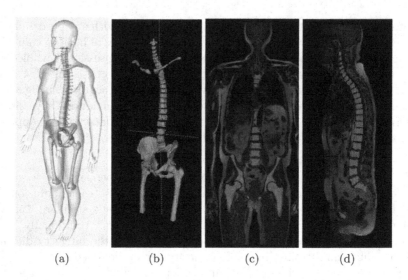

(a)   (b)   (c)   (d)

Fig. 3. (a) Anatomical reference from Bio Digital [13]. (b) Volume rendering from manual segmentation. (c) Coronal and (d) sagittal slice of a whole-body T_1 image in overlay with bone segmentation mask (yellow). (Color figure online)

2.4 Validation

Two validation criteria were used to asses similarity of skeletal intensity profiles between a reference baseline and target follow-up image.

Mean Absolute Difference: Corresponding voxel intensities were compared and summed into a mean absolute difference (MAD) value

$$MAD = \frac{\sum_x |f(x) - g'((\mathcal{T}_\mu(x))|}{N},\tag{4}$$

where, $f(x)$ and $g'(\mathcal{T}_\mu(x))$ are image intensities of the reference and spatially registered - intensity standardized target image in the corresponding voxel location x and N is a number of image voxels.

Kullback-Leibler Divergence: We have implemented the Kullback-Leibler divergence (KL) representing a distance measure between two discrete probability distributions (histograms)

$$KL_D = \sum_i P(i) log \frac{Q(i)}{P(i)},\tag{5}$$

where, $P(i)$ and $Q(i)$ are discrete probability distributions of a reference and standardized image at histogram bin i.

We can assume that if different tissue classes cover the same intensity range in both volumes, the histograms of a reference and target whole-body image will be as similar as possible, representing KL value close to zero.

Since not all of the data proved to be normally distributed ($p > 0.05$, Shapiro-Wilk Normality Test [16]), the Wilcoxon two-tailed, signed-rank test was used to investigate statistical significance of differences in validation criteria values between the non-standardized image and each of the registration strategies separately. The p-value used for the statistical significance test was equal to 0.05.

3 Results

All proposed intensity standardization methods were quantitatively validated and compared to a spatially registered and non-standardized whole-body image pair, representing a baseline value. Results of the validation criteria representing intensity standardization performance between baseline whole-body image and follow-up whole-body image, averaged over all subjects used, are presented in Table 2. Figure 4 shows the influence of the spatial registration and intensity standardization on baseline and follow-up image skeleton similarity. Figure 5 shows whole-body T_1 and DWI baseline and follow-up images before and after intensity standardization displayed with the same window and level setting. A sample T_1 functional response map indicating metastatic bone disease progression is shown in Fig. 6.

Table 2. Evaluation metrics averaged over 10 whole-body image pairs of T_1 and DWI modalities for the proposed methods ($\pm$ standard deviation). The best performing strategy in terms of average for each criteria is highlighted in bold. Statistical significance for each registration strategy and evaluation criterion, when compared to unregistered raw images is marked with an asterix (*).

	MAD	KL divergence
No standardization	143.20 ± 126.67	0.540 ± 0.520
Method 1	76.15 ± 91.49	0.540 ± 0.520
Method 2	69.27 ± 81.77	0.468 ± 0.678
Method 2.1	**49.29 ± 50.68***	**0.095 ± 0.122***
Method 3	64.86 ± 60.22*	0.165 ± 0.169*
Method 3.1	64.32 ± 74.37*	0.484 ± 0.399

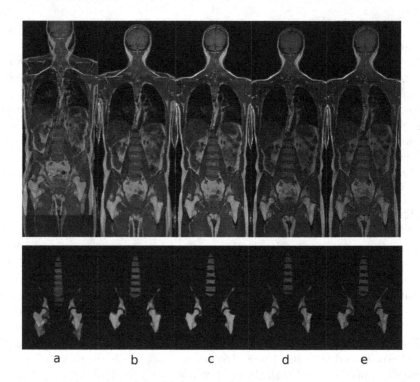

a   b   c   d   e

Fig. 4. Coronal overlay view of whole-body T_1 image (top) with extracted skeleton (bottom). Pink and green colours indicate intensity difference. **(a)** Raw images, **(b)** result after rigid registration, **(c)** result after deformable registration, **(d)** result after deformable registration with linear scaling of intensities (Method 1), **(e)** result after deformable registration with intensity standardization (Method 2.1). (Color figure online)

3.1   Computation Times

Processing was performed using a 2.5 GHz Intel® Core® i7-4870HQ processor and 16 GB RAM. Spatial registration inducing preprocessing steps and image re-sampling took around 30 min for an image pair. The entire standardization procedure (single threaded execution) for method 1 and all variations of method 2, took around 1 min. Method 3 with an execution time equal to 30 min, is considerably more expensive due to the deformable histogram registration and a higher number of intensity transformations equal to the size of the 1D deformation field.

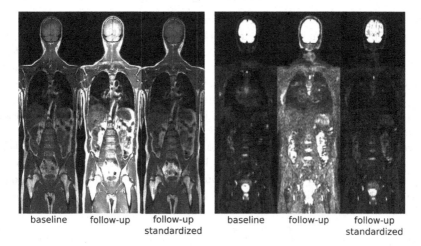

Fig. 5. Whole-body T_1 (left) and DWI (right) baseline and follow-up images before and after intensity standardization (Method 2.1). Images have been spatially registered. All images are displayed with the same window and level setting.

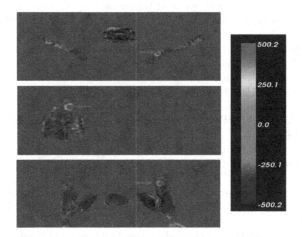

Fig. 6. From top to bottom: axial, sagittal and coronal view of functional response map calculated on T_1 intensity standardized image showing left upper pelvis with a visible progression of focal bone metastasis (red arrow). (Color figure online)

4   Discussion and Conclusion

In this work we investigated several strategies for intra-patient whole-body intensity standardization of skeleton profiles. Five different intensity standardization methods were compared and their performance was validated. Additionally, the use of spatial registration between the baseline and follow-up volumes, allowed for the introduction of strong validation criterion based on direct intensity difference - mean absolute difference of skeleton intensity profiles. The piecewise linear method using the masked tissue of interest (Method 2.1) performed better than other evaluated methods, showing high stability and robustness of performance. Slightly worse performance of masked 1D deformable method (Method 3.1) might be caused by the limited amount of image information which corrupts the performance of deformable registration algorithms and the over-fitting of the match of the intensity profiles. Intensity standardization algorithms can be applied to any other tissue of interest if a specific mask representing a tissue type is provided.

Accurate intensity standardization of intra-patient MRI whole-body skeleton profiles, opens opportunities for whole-body quantitative follow-up, cohort comparison studies and functional response maps for non-quantitative modalities, considerably simplifying extraction of relevant quantitative information for healthy and disease.

References

1. Baur-Melnyk, A., Buhmann, S., Dürr, H., Reiser, M.: Role of MRI for the diagnosis and prognosis of multiple myeloma. Eur. J. Radiol. **55**(1), 56–63 (2005)
2. Blackledge, M.D., et al.: Assessment of treatment response by total tumor volume and global apparent diffusion coefficient using diffusion-weighted MRI in patients with metastatic bone disease: a feasibility study. PLoS ONE **9**(4), e91779 (2014)
3. Darge, K., Jaramillo, D., Siegel, M.J.: Whole-body MRI in children: current status and future applications. Eur. J. Radiol. **68**(2), 289–298 (2008)
4. Fedorov, A., et al.: 3D slicer as an image computing platform for the quantitative imaging network. Magn. Reson. Imaging **30**(9), 1323–1341 (2012)
5. Jäger, F., Hornegger, J.: Nonrigid registration of joint histograms for intensity standardization in magnetic resonance imaging. IEEE Trans. Med. Imaging **28**(1), 137–150 (2009)
6. Karlsson, A., et al.: Automatic and quantitative assessment of regional muscle volume by multi-atlas segmentation using whole-body water-fat MRI. J. Magn. Reson. Imaging **41**(6), 1558–1569 (2015)
7. Klein, S., Staring, M., Murphy, K., Viergever, M.A., Pluim, J.P.: Elastix: a toolbox for intensity-based medical image registration. IEEE Trans. Med. Imaging **29**(1), 196–205 (2010)
8. Lecouvet, F.E., et al.: Can whole-body magnetic resonance imaging with diffusion-weighted imaging replace Tc 99m bone scanning and computed tomography for single-step detection of metastases in patients with high-risk prostate cancer? Eur. Urol. **62**(1), 68–75 (2012)
9. Maes, F., Collignon, A., Vandermeulen, D., Marchal, G., Suetens, P.: Multimodality image registration by maximization of mutual information. IEEE Trans. Med. Imaging **16**(2), 187–198 (1997)
10. Nyúl, L.G., Udupa, J.K., Zhang, X.: New variants of a method of MRI scale standardization. IEEE Trans. Med. Imaging **19**(2), 143–150 (2000)
11. Padhani, A.R., Makris, A., Gall, P., Collins, D.J., Tunariu, N., de Bono, J.S.: Therapy monitoring of skeletal metastases with whole-body diffusion MRI. J. Magn. Reson. Imaging **39**(5), 1049–1078 (2014)
12. Pasoglou, V., et al.: Whole-body 3D T1-weighted MR imaging in patients with prostate cancer: feasibility and evaluation in screening for metastatic disease. Radiology **275**(1), 155–166 (2014)

13. Qualter, J., et al.: The biodigital human: a web-based 3D platform for medical visualization and education. Stud. Health Technol. Inform. **173**, 359–361 (2012)
14. Robitaille, N., Mouiha, A., Crépeault, B., Valdivia, F., Duchesne, S.: Tissue-based MRI intensity standardization: application to multicentric datasets. J. Biomed. Imaging **2012**, 4 (2012)
15. Rueckert, D., Sonoda, L.I., Hayes, C., Hill, D.L., Leach, M.O., Hawkes, D.J.: Non-rigid registration using free-form deformations: application to breast MR images. IEEE Trans. Med. Imaging **18**(8), 712–721 (1999)
16. Shapiro, S.S., Wilk, M.B.: An analysis of variance test for normality (complete samples). Biometrika **52**(3/4), 591–611 (1965)
17. Strand, R., et al.: A concept for holistic whole body MRI data analysis Imiomics. PloS one **12**(2), e0169966 (2017)
18. Tustison, N.J., et al.: N4ITK: improved N3 bias correction. IEEE Trans. Med. Imaging **29**(6), 1310–1320 (2010)

Towards a Deformable Multi-surface Approach to Ligamentous Spine Models for Predictive Simulation-Based Scoliosis Surgery Planning

Michel A. Audette[1(✉)], Jerome Schmid[2,3], Craig Goodmurphy[4],
Michael Polanco[1], Sebastian Bawab[1], Austin Tapp[1],
and H. Sheldon St-Clair[5]

[1] Old Dominion University, Norfolk, VA, USA
maudette@odu.edu
[2] Haute Ecole de Santé, Geneva, Switzerland
[3] HES-SO University of Applied Sciences and Arts Western Switzerland,
Delémont, Switzerland
[4] Eastern Virginia Medical School, Norfolk, VA, USA
[5] Children's Hospital of the King's Daughters, Norfolk, VA, USA

Abstract. Scoliosis correction surgery is typically a highly invasive procedure that involves either an anterior or posterior release, which respectively entail the resection of ligaments and bone facets from the front or back of the spine, in order to make it sufficiently compliant to enable the correction of the deformity. In light of progress in other areas of surgery in minimally invasive therapies, orthopedic surgeons have begun envisioning computer simulation-assisted planning that could answer unprecedented what-if questions. This paper presents preliminary steps taken towards simulation-based surgery planning that will provide answers as to how much anterior or posterior release is truly necessary, provided we also establish the amplitude of surgical forces involved in corrective surgery. This question motivates us to pursue a medical image-based anatomical modeling pipeline that can support personalized finite elements simulation, based on models of the spine that not only feature vertebrae and inter-vertebral discs (IVDs), but also descriptive ligament models. This paper suggests a way of proceeding, based on the application of deformable multi-surface Simplex model applied to a CAD-based representation of the spine that makes explicit all spinal ligaments, along with vertebrae and IVDs. It presents a preliminary model-based segmentation study whereby Simplex meshes of CAD vertebrae are registered to the subject's corresponding vertebrae in CT data, which then drives ligament and IVD model registration by aggregation of neighboring vertebral transformations. This framework also anticipates foreseen improvements in MR imaging that could achieve better contrasts in ligamentous tissues in the future.

Keywords: Scoliosis surgery · Surgery planning · Finite elements simulation · Spinal ligaments · Minimally invasive surgery · Surface meshing · Mesh repair

© Springer Nature Switzerland AG 2019
G. Zheng et al. (Eds.): CSI 2018, LNCS 11397, pp. 90–102, 2019.
https://doi.org/10.1007/978-3-030-13736-6_8

1   Introduction

1.1   Background – Scoliosis

Scoliosis is a medical condition in which a person's spinal axis has a three-dimensional deviation, which viewed from the rear can resemble an "S" or a "C" rather than a straight line. Scoliosis is defined as a spinal curvature of more than 10° to the right or left in the coronal plane. Deformity may also exist in the sagittal plane. Its causes include neuromuscular problems, genetic conditions, and limb length inequality. Scoliosis is typically classified as either congenital (caused by vertebral anomalies present at birth), idiopathic (cause unknown), or secondary to a primary condition. X-rays are usually taken to assess the scoliosis curves and the kyphosis and lordosis, convex and concave curvatures in the sagittal plane that can also individuals with scoliosis. Instrumented scoliosis surgery was first performed in the 1960s [1], subsequent to which, device and technique modifications since then have led to improved surgical results. The goals of surgical management of adolescent idiopathic scoliosis (AIS) include maintaining coronal and sagittal alignment, producing level shoulders, correcting deformity, and saving motion segments [2]. Classification systems for AIS are useful for surgical planning and for comparing postoperative results. However, choosing optimal fusion levels remains challenging; in a study by Lenke, an average of five different proximal fusion levels and four different distal fusion levels were identified in AIS cases presented to 28 surgeons [3].

Computer simulation of scoliosis treatment can provide an efficient, risk-free means of finding the optimum among competing therapeutic approaches. The main objective of this project will be to predict the amplitude of the forces needed to correct the scoliotic spine, for example to ensure adequate fixation. However, a long-term objective is to provide the orthopedic surgery community with a predictive planning tool that enables the exploration of what-if scenarios by clinicians both as individuals and as a community, which will likely lead to greater consensus for various categories of scoliotic deformity as well as for other orthopedics cases (herniated disc, trauma, and so on) in the long term.

The proposed study describes a first instantiation of a deformable multi-surface approach to constructing a ligamentous patient-specific anatomy; it is presented as a preliminary result that will be improved upon through an on-going approach founded on multi-material surface extraction, whose objective will ultimately be to preserve shared boundaries (flush surfaces) where appropriate. The main objective of this study is to demonstrate the feasibility of using the model-image transformations undergone by vertebral surfaces of a descriptive spine model, drawn with CAD software by an anatomist, to anchor the nonrigid transformation of neighboring soft tissues (IVDs, ligaments). Moreover, these soft-tissue transformations may be further refined by medical images if adequate contrast is available, particularly as imaging techniques (MRI pulse sequences and high-field imaging) evolve to capture greater anatomical details.

1.2   Limitations in Current Scoliosis Surgery Planning – Impetus for Minimally Invasive Approach

For many scoliosis cases, the rigidity of the deformity cannot be overcome enough to achieve satisfactory correction, without using measures to make the spine more compliant. In these cases, a release procedure, either anterior or posterior, is used to render the spine more flexible and enable correction, albeit at the cost of a more complex and extensive procedure, as shown in Fig. 1. In an anterior release, as in Fig. 1a, intervertebral disc (IVD) tissue is removed from the front. Furthermore, the anterior longitudinal ligament is cut at each relevant IVD. Alternately, posterior column osteotomy, of Smith-Petersen or Ponte type, involves the posterior removal of ligament and bone, as in Fig. 1b, including parts of the spinous process and facets to partially correct scoliosis. Subsequently, the surgeon inserts pedicle screws, typically in both vertebral pedicles, one of which will be used to cup a portion of a curved rod that mirrors the deformation of the spine of the patient. This curved rod has a personalized shape, which can be produced during the procedure by the surgeon himself, so as to correspond to the scoliotic curvature of the patient. Once the curved rod is inserted in all of the corresponding pedicle anchors, the surgeon imparts a 90-degree rotation to this curved rod, which effectively straightens the spine, as seen in Fig. 2. Typically, this correction requires a significant amount of force, even after anterior/posterior release, and necessitates a pair of vice-grip-like surgical pliers to lock onto two points on the curved rod. If the amplitude of corrective forces were known prior to surgery, surgical workflow would be improved, the patient would spend less time in the operating room, while limiting anterior and posterior release procedures to a minimum and generally facilitating their planning. While finite-elements-based biomechanical studies in surgery are not new, they emphasize pedicle screw insertion mechanics [5, 6]. Meanwhile, patient- specific anatomical models that account for interaction between vertebrae, bound to each other by ligaments, are generally not found in the literature or in clinical practice.

As a result, existing work in surgery planning or simulation does not provide a surgeon with an estimate of the amplitude of corrective forces involved in scoliosis surgery.

These limitations of state-of-the-art surgery simulation and planning have two main root causes. First, spinal ligaments are not easily delineated in MRI or CT: these tissues exhibit little contrast in relation to other soft tissues nearby. Second, even if one were able to identify these tissues (through segmentation), these tissue blobs would need to be decomposed into elements (by volumetric meshing), such as tetrahedral or hexahedra: this multi-material volumetric meshing is not done adequately in the current state of the art, namely in a manner that produces high-fidelity patient-specific models.

Recently, research on the large-scale compliance of the spine has been published in the biomechanics literature [9]. However, in the absence of a digital atlas of spinal ligaments, biomechanists have to resort to modeling ligaments as a set of one-dimensional rods whose anchor points are imposed by hand, as depicted in Fig. 3, the limitations of which are described in detail in the Methods section.

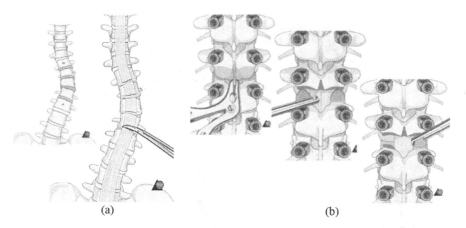

(a)   (b)

Fig. 1. (a) Anterior release: discectomy and resection of annulus of every intervertebral disk within the instrumented area: the annulus is incised from the lateral aspect of the spine, the disk is removed with curettes and rongeurs. The anterior longitudinal ligament is cut; the posterior annulus may be removed. (b) Posterior column osteotomy (left to right). First, resect the inferior aspect of the spinous process, followed by removal of the interspinous ligament with a rongeur. Second, remove 3–5 mm of inferior aspect of inferior facet joint at each level of the planned fusion with an osteotome. The ligamentum flavum is removed with a Kerrison rongeur while avoiding to penetrate deeply against the dura. Last, a Kerrison rongeur is utilized to remove the superior portion of the superior articular facet. Reproduced with permission from AO Foundation [4].

With the proposed anatomical modeling approach, founded on a deformable multi-surface model fitted to an anatomist-drawn Computer-Aided Design (CAD) template, we have the means to produce patient-specific finite element studies for a number of applications in orthopedics, emphasizing in this project the estimation of corrective forces in scoliosis surgery. This anatomical modeling technique, which addresses both segmentation and meshing, warps the CAD-based anatomical template to any individual's CT/MR image dataset and can guide subsequent multi-tissue high-fidelity two-stage tetrahedral meshing [10]. This two-stage tetrahedralization approach consists of (i) a *surfacic* first stage, founded on a discrete deformable surface model [11], which produces a controlled-resolution high-fidelity triangulated boundary, followed by (ii) *volumetric* second stage: controlled-resolution variational tetrahedral meshing [12] (found in CGAL [13]). The latter stage uses as input a prescribed triangulated mesh boundary resulting from the first stage. *The deformable multi-surface model computation effectively integrates the segmentation and the first stage of the meshing in one step.* For validation, we also planning some cadaveric image studies, featuring point clouds identified by an anatomist and coinciding with the boundaries of the ligaments.

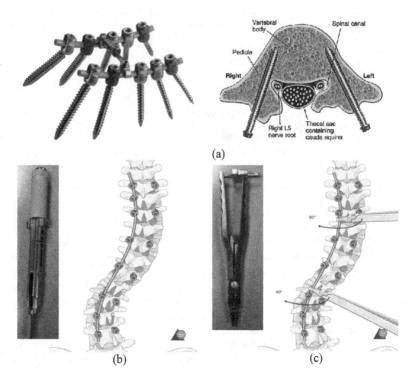

(a)

(b)   (c)

Fig. 2. Technical aspects of surgical scoliosis correction. (a) Pedicle screw-anchored rod fixation: (left) assembly featuring inserted rods; (right) correct screw insertion into vertebral pedicles and body [7, 8]. (b) Reduction procedure whereby a rod is inserted into the tops of the screws; inset: reduction tower for rod insertion [4]. (c) 90-degree rotation that performs the correction; inset: pliers used for rod rotation [4]. Figures b and c reproduced with permission; Copyright by AO Foundation, Switzerland [4].

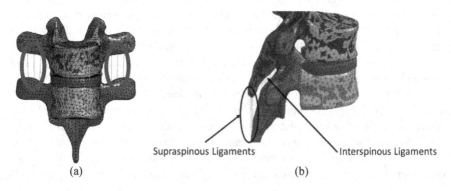

Supraspinous Ligaments   Interspinous Ligaments

(a)   (b)

Fig. 3. Motivation for an automatic ligamentous spine model computation: manual identification of ligamentous constraints for finite element studies (ongoing work). (a) Intratransverse ligaments (brown threads). (b) Supraspinous and interspinous ligaments (both labeled). (Color figure online)

2 Methods

2.1 Anatomist-Drawn Ligamentous CAD Model of the Spine

The cornerstone of our approach to achieving descriptive personalized anatomical models of the spine is a CAD model that is commercially available through the TurboSquid website [14]. The justification for using such a model is that it is virtually impossible to volumetrically reconstruct the spinal ligaments from current routine imaging modalities, either CT or MRI-based, using voxel-based segmentation techniques. The descriptiveness required of the anatomy necessarily imposes a top-down, model-based segmentation approach, which naturally maps to a multi-surface anatomical atlas.

Moreover, in existing efforts to run finite element studies of the ligamentous spine, while factoring in the constraining effect of the ligaments (Fig. 3), the current means of representing the ligaments is limited to a terse representation based on a set of linear constraints that are drawn by hand from one vertebral surface point to its opposing surface landmark: each ligament is thus approximated as a simple collection of 1D springs or stiff rods. We argue that, while this current approach is certainly an improvement over an entirely untethered spine model, *it is potentially limiting in relation to the complexity of the 3D ligament geometry and onerous in terms of user interaction, as is visible in Fig. 3b in interspinous ligaments in particular.*

Moreover, should there be rheological studies published on spinal ligaments, which could be used to populate the material properties of such a finite element model of the spine, it would prove difficult to relate a small set of 1D springs to such properties acquired by stress-strain experiments on a shell-like structure. In contrast, these properties would naturally feed right into an anatomical model that faithfully replicates the curviplanar or volumetric structure, depending on the thickness of the ligament. In short, *while manual rod/spring delineation is vital to tethering the spine, it underrepresents the complexity of the constraining ligamentous geometry*, which may have a dire impact on the fidelity of the finite element studies.

2.2 Using Descriptive CAD Models for Segmentation – Deformable Multi-surface Models

As is true of all CAD drawings, the TurboSquid spine model (Fig. 4) is a collection of polygons, typically 2D B-spline quadrilateral patches, which are easily converted to a triangulated surface: each quad patch is bisected into two triangles. Moreover, as can be seen in Fig. 5 and used extensively in our research, a triangulated surface can be used to initialize a deformable surface model, such as the Simplex [11], through geometric duality. The latter represents the second foundational aspect of our work:

CAD B-spline surface → CAD triangulated surface
(→ Watertight triangulated surface) →Deformable Simplex model.

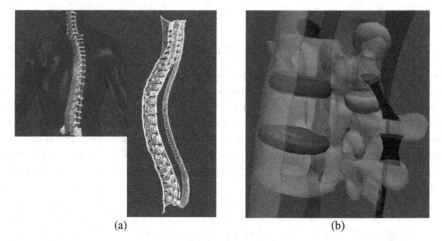

(a)   (b)

Fig. 4. Anatomist-drawn ligamentous CAD model of the spine. (a) Spine model displayed in its native Maya environment. Insert top left: surface rendering of the models of spline-based spine and ligament anatomical surfaces in Maya format, overlaid on translucent body surface. Right: wireframe rendering of the ligament model. (b) Close-up of a subset of the anatomy, converted to triangulated surfaces (stored in .obj format), featuring the following components as visualized with Paraview: C7, T1 and T2 vertebrae (white translucent), C7-T1 and T1-T2 IVDs (purple), local ligaments: intertransverse (dark green), interspinous (cyan), capsulary (orange), and ligamentum flavum (pink); ligaments spanning several vertebrae: anterior (yellow translucent) and posterior (rust) longitudinal ligaments, nuchal (dark red, spanning C1-C6) and supraspinous (dark blue, spanning C7-sacrum) ligaments. (Color figure online)

This recipe, although simple, is fundamental and surprisingly absent in the literature:
this methodology suggests that we use an anatomist's CAD drawing of an arbitrary anatomy as a foundation for a deformable multi-surface model-based segmentation.

Although the results presented in this paper build on a naïve single-surface Simplex model, such as developed by Delingette [11], it is feasible to transition to a multi-surface approach [15, 16], which will be integrated into the second version of our methodology. The Simplex is a discrete deformable mesh model, characterized by a set of vertices linked by edges, and governed by a Newtonian model of vertex motion:

$$m\frac{d^2P_i}{dt^2} = -\gamma\frac{dP_i}{dt} + \alpha F_{int} + \beta F_{ext} \tag{1}$$

where m and γ represent vertex mass and damping, and the latter two terms are sums of internal and external forces. Moreover, an N-Simplex is a mesh where every vertex is linked to $N + 1$ neighbors by edges. The 2-Simplex thus exhibits 3-connectivity, as shown in Fig. 5a. Note the geometric duality between the 2-Simplex mesh in black and triangulated mesh in blue. The external force F_{ext} includes an image force that binds the model to anatomical boundaries of interest, typically characterized by strong gradient magnitude in a linear search space along the direction normal to each vertex.

There are two options for extending this single-surface deformable model to espouse multiple anatomical boundaries, and such an extension is foreseen in the near future. Gilles' multi-surface model featuring a static collision detection between individual surfaces [15]. Haq has integrated this multi-surface model with shape statistics force for spine applications. Rashid's multi-surface Simplex model emphasizes shared boundaries based on multi-material surface extraction [17], which was used to achieve a lightweight deformable atlas of basal ganglia for efficient intraoperative-MRI-based guidance in robotic deep-brain stimulation. The latter multi-surface approach is advantageous in that it produces models of the weight-bearing anatomy with flush surfaces where needed, which is highly desirable in orthopedic finite elements applications.

It is worth noting that there are numerous resources available online to facilitate the computation of a watertight triangulated surface mesh, in the event that the surface model is derived from a voxel-based atlas by surface extraction (e.g. available on Paraview) or that there is a manifold inconsistency in the CAD model. Conversely, all it takes to throw off the geometric duality of the triangulated surface with the Simplex mesh is one hole or one non-manifold edge, whereby the deformable surface model is doomed to failure. Based on the recipe suggested in [18], Poisson Surface Reconstruction can be useful in correcting small surface inconsistencies (non-manifold edges, inconsistent surface normals, etc.), while Quadric Edge Collapse decimation enables us to control surface mesh resolution while preserving topology. Both surface mesh processing algorithms are found in MeshLab [19]. In the case of the CAD model described above, most surface models were a watertight collection of quadrilaterals that could be diagonalized to produce a triangulated surface (through MeshLab's triangular mesh conversion). In the absence of a statistical pose model that can simplify the registration of each vertebra, we opted for a homologous point-based registration using 17 anatomical landmarks, identified using Slicer 3D planning software [20], which could reliably be located both on the vertebral model surface and in the target image. A few models, namely the capsular ligament, contained holes: plugging such openings in an unsupervised manner is the specialty of MeshFix [21].

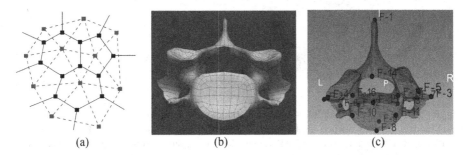

(a)   (b)   (c)

Fig. 5. Computation of CAD-based Simplex vertebral model. (a) 2-Simplex surface mesh model in black, with dual triangulation in blue. (b) C7 vertebral CAD model, depicting B-spline quadrilaterals. (c) Triangulated surface, used to initialize Simplex by duality, with typical landmark configuration for initializing a vertebral registration by homologous point pairs. (Color figure online)

In fact, for this simple proof of concept, the target image was taken from the SpineWeb database and featured segmented vertebrae, however it was still vital to warp the CAD model's vertebrae to the SpineWeb model. Our goal with this exercise is not to innovate on vertebral segmentation, but to demonstrate the merit of the chain effect whereby vertebral model transformations, which are unambiguously determined by sharp contrasts in a medical image, particularly CT, are aggregated and used to drive the registration of nearby soft-tissue structures. This is achieved while preserving the neighborhood topology throughout; ultimately, using contiguity with unambiguously registered vertebral surfaces to constrain the positioning of soft tissue models.

The transformation used to initialize the Simplex warping is itself a simpler non-rigid mapping based on homologous point pairs, namely the Thin-Plate Spline (TPS) transformation [22]. This method leads to a stable elastic transformation that maps a CAD vertebral surface model to the target boundary in the CT image, as can be seen from the overlay of warped CAD model surface over a surface extracted from the known boundary of the SpineWeb segmentation. Alternately, we can use an Iterative Closest Point method to establish the vertebral registration that will serve as anchor for the soft tissues, if we have a starting point of known anatomical boundaries of voxel-based segmentation. Figure 6 depicts a typical result of a TPS-initialized vertebral surface model, after 600 iterations of the Simplex, overlaid in red on the known boundary of a SpineWeb model's C7 cervical vertebra, depicted in white. The set of such vertebral registrations will then serve to orient the soft-tissue surfaces attached to neighboring vertebrae. This vertebral registration is not the main aspect of the inno-vation: it serves as a foundational set of pitons we use to anchor our ascent, so to speak.

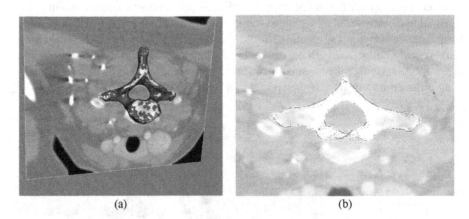

(a)   (b)

Fig. 6. TPS-initialized, Simplex-mesh-based model-to-target image registration of vertebral CAD models. (a) Red warped model overlaid on white gold-standard surface from SpineWeb, with 3D-mapped 2D axial slice in background. (b) 2D contour depicting planar intersections of surfaces in a, mapped to red contour and purple gold-standard points respectively. (Color figure online)

2.3 Exploiting Well-Defined Vertebral Transformations to Drive Ambiguous Ligament and IVD Model Registration

The stable nonrigid registration of the CAD vertebral models can be aggregated to produce a putative registration of the IVD and ligaments, in a number of ways. One option would have been to distill each vertebral elastic registration into rotation and translation parameters that can be averaged or weighted according to proximity if dealing with a structure in between two vertebrae, and then use static collision detection to nudge overlapping surfaces away from each other. Ideally, if any image contrast information is available, if for progress is made with high-field MR scanners for example, image gradients could be used to finalize the image boundaries. Of course, one of the advantages of shared-surface boundary-preserving meshing is that vertebral surfaces will have direct implications for the boundaries of soft-tissue structures in contact with them. Alternately, as currently pursued here, a subsample of warped vertebral model points can be leveraged to determine a local TPS transformation that is in turn applied to a local neighborhood; where two warped vertebral models abut, they contribute to the local elastic transformation that is applied to soft-tissue surfaces affixed to them in the CAD model. Typical results are shown in the following section.

3 Results and Discussion

Currently, our validation is qualitative rather than quantitative, due to the difficulty of obtaining ground truth expert segmentations of the ligaments, which after all are elusive in existing CT or MRI alone. We can point to qualitative results that appear promising to an orthopedic surgeon on the team, as shown in Fig. 7. This figure depicts surface-rendered visualizations and rasterized images of planar intersections of the warped CAD model overlaid on the corresponding CT plane.

In fact, the planned validation strategy can briefly be described as follows. This validation methodology is currently under development through the efforts of the anatomists on the team. As shown in Fig. 8, the validation will exploit cadaveric imaging studies that integrate, on the one hand, high-resolution CT and MRI image acquisitions, interspersed with expert suturing of radiolucent thread at the surface of these ligaments, producing point cloud sets that will coincide with the boundaries, for comparison with those produced by the warped multi-surface model. These cadaveric studies could also lead to a shape statistics model, whose integration with multi-surface Simplex was shown by Haq et al. [16].

As mentioned above, this work is still in a nascent stage, but will soon integrate further surface meshing innovations. We could employ the static collision detection between neighboring surfaces to prevent overlap, as developed by Gilles [15] and also applied by Haq to the lumbar spine [16]. However, this implementation only prevents spatial overlap between two neighboring surfaces: *it does not in any way ensure that these surfaces should be flush with one another*. A better approach has been proposed by Rashid [17], as depicted in Fig. 9 below: *multi-material surface extraction* leads to a triangulated *multi-surface complex with shared boundaries*: this multi-surface model can then be converted to a deformable multi-surface Simplex model by geometric

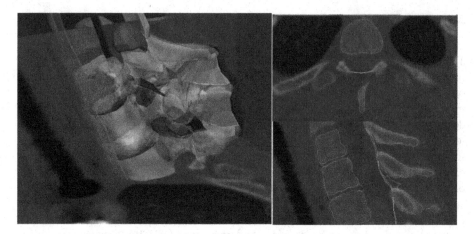

Fig. 7. Left: MITK Workbench [23] scene with registered semitransparent vertebrae C7, T1 and T2, with two IVDs sandwiched between them and all ligament models of Fig. 4b, defined in relation to these vertebrae and rendered with the same color codes. Right top and bottom: axial and sagittal planes featuring colored contours coinciding with intersecting surface models. Right: 3D multi-planar view featuring embedded registered surfaces. (Color figure online)

duality, which then allows us to warp the anatomy to the target image, while continuing to enforce shared boundaries. *With a shared-boundary deformable multi-surface model, IVD-vertebra and ligament-vertebra interfaces will thus remain in perfect contact throughout the deformation.*

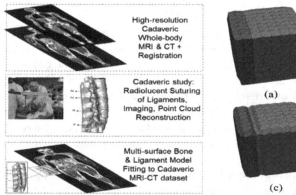

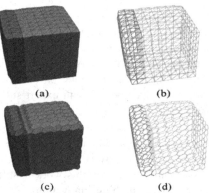

Fig. 8. Planned validation study founded on cadaveric MR, CT and radiolucent suturing-based point cloud acquisition, coincident with ligament boundaries.

Fig. 9. Planned multi-material shared-boundary multi-surface model. (a-b) Synthetic triangulated multi-material boundary, surface and wireframe-rendered. (c-d) Dual shared-boundary simplex, (c) surface and (d) wireframe-rendered. Reproduced from [17].

Given that the starting point is a *collection of individual surfaces, with tiny spaces between them,* the implementation of a multi-material surface extraction will require a competitive Fast Marching method-based multi-front propagation of the various boundaries within a fine-resolution image volume, to flag overlaps and seal small "air pockets". Surfaces that should anatomically be in contact will then exhibit airtight contiguity in labeled fine-resolution image volumes. In turn, this airtight digital atlas of the ligamentous spine will be input to Rashid's shared-boundary-preserving multi-surface extraction. One aspect of this method that requires further work is a decimation technique for the multi-material Simplex model, which preserves double vertices and edges on both sides of the interface. This decimation is needed to produce a suitably sparse multi-surface complex that affords a robust, coarse-to-fine registration to the target image.

Last, the pre-Simplex TPS transformation exhibits undulations, which is typical of an interpolation of this nature. It is likely that a regularized approach, or alternately a thin plate-based approximation, would be less prone to this oscillatory behavior.

4   Conclusions

This paper presented a novel approach to producing personalized anatomical models of the spine that emphasize ligaments, in conjunction with the development of a finite elements simulation-based scoliosis surgery planning. While the meshing methodology is currently well proven, the application of anatomist-drawn CAD models is new and broadly applicable to orthopedic surgery planning in general: knee, shoulder, pelvis, and so on, provided that sufficiently descriptive and faithful CAD models of the relevant anatomy be available. This method also does not preclude further image-mediated refinements in the event that high-contrast delineation of the ligaments becomes available in MRI: the application of shared-boundary multi-surface Simplex models to tracking 3D image gradients has been demonstrated in deep brain data by Rashid [17].

References

1. Harrington, P.R.: Treatment of scoliosis: correction and internal fixation by spine instrumentation. J. Bone Joint Surg. Am. **44**(A), 591–610 (1962)
2. Trobisch, P.D., Ducoffe, A.R., Lonner, B.S., Errico, T.J.: Choosing fusion levels in adolescent idiopathic scoliosis. J. Am. Acad. Orthop. Surg. **21**(9), 519–528 (2013). https://doi.org/10.5435/jaaos-21-09-519
3. Lenke, L.G., et al.: Multisurgeon assessment of surgical decision-making in adolescent idiopathic scoliosis: curve classification, operative approach, and fusion levels. Spine **26**(21), 2347–2353 (2001). (Phila Pa 1976)
4. AO Foundation. Adolescent Idiopathic Scoliosis Lenke 6 - Posterior Screws - With direct vertebral body derotation. www2.aofoundation.org
5. Cho, W., Cho, S.K., Wu, C.: The biomechanics of pedicle screw-based instrumentation. J. Bone Joint Surg. Br. **92**(8), 1061–1065 (2010). https://doi.org/10.1302/0301-620X.92B8.24237

6. Bianco, R.J., Aubin, C.E., Mac-Thiong, J.M., Wagnac, E., Eng, P., Arnoux, P.J.: Pedicle screw fixation under non-axial loads: a cadaveric study. Spine (Phila Pa 1976), 15 October 2015. (Epub ahead of print)

7. Renovis. S100 Pedicle Screw System. http://www.renovis-surgical.com/2011/09/s100-pedicle-screw-system/

8. Neurology Update. Making Sure Pedicle Screws are Correctly Placed During Spine Surgery. https://mmcneuro.wordpress.com/2013/02/

9. Hortin, M.S., Bowden, A.E.: Quantitative comparison of ligament formulation and pre-strain in finite element analysis of the human lumbar spine. Comput. Methods Biomech. Biomed. Engin. **19**(14), 1505–15018 (2016)

10. Audette, M.A., et al.: A Topologically faithful, tissue-guided, spatially varying meshing strategy for computing patient-specific head models for endoscopic pituitary surgery simulation. J. Comput. Aided Surg. **12**(1), 43–52 (2007)

11. Delingette, H.: General object reconstruction based on simplex meshes. Int. J. Comput. Vis. **32**(2), 111–146 (1999)

12. Alliez, P., Cohen-Steiner, D., Yvinec, M., Desbrun, M.: Variational tetrahedral meshing. ACM Trans. Graph **24**(3), 617–625 (2005). https://doi.org/10.1145/1073204.1073238

13. CGAL. The Computational Geometry Algorithms Library. http://www.cgal.org/

14. TurboSquid. TurboSquid 3D Spine Models. https://www.turbosquid.com/Search/3D-Models/spine

15. Gilles, B., Magnenat-Thalmann, N.: Musculoskeletal MRI segmentation using multi-resolution simplex meshes with medial representations. Med. Image Anal. **14**(3), 291–302 (2010)

16. Haq, R., Cates, J., Besachio, D.A., Borgie, R.C., Audette, M.A.: Statistical shape model construction of lumbar vertebrae and intervertebral discs in segmentation for discectomy surgery simulation. In: Vrtovec, T., et al. (eds.) CSI 2015. LNCS, vol. 9402, pp. 85–96. Springer, Cham (2016). https://doi.org/10.1007/978-3-319-41827-8_8

17. Rashid, T., Sultana, S., Fischer, G.S., Pilitsis, J., Audette, M.A.: Deformable multi-material 2-simplex surface mesh for intraoperative MRI-ready surgery planning and simulation, with deep-brain stimulation applications. In: Cardoso, M.J., et al. (eds.) BIVPCS/POCUS-2017. LNCS, vol. 10549, pp. 94–102. Springer, Cham (2017). https://doi.org/10.1007/978-3-319-67552-7_12

18. Meshlab. Meshlab Stuff - Practical Mesh Processing Experiments. http://meshlabstuff.blogspot.com/2010/07/remeshing-and-texturing-1.html

19. MeshLab. MeshLab. http://www.meshlab.net/

20. Slicer 3D. Slicer 4.6 released. https://www.slicer.org/

21. MeshFix. MeshFix SourceForge repository. https://sourceforge.net/projects/meshfix/

22. Bookstein, F.L.: Principal Warps: thin-plate splines and the decomposition of deformations. IEEE Trans. Pattern Anal. Mach. Intell. **11**(6), 567–585 (1989). https://doi.org/10.1109/34.24792

23. MITK. Medical Imaging Interaction Toolkit (MITK) - Downloads. http://mitk.org/wiki/Downloads

IVDM3Seg Challenge

Intervertebral Disc Segmentation Using Mathematical Morphology—A CNN-Free Approach

Edwin Carlinet[✉] and Thierry Géraud

EPITA Research and Development Laboratory (LRDE),
Le Kremlin-Bicêtre, France
edwin.carlinet@lrde.epita.fr

Abstract. In the context of the challenge of "automatic InterVertebral Disc (IVD) localization and segmentation from 3D multi-modality MR images" that took place at MICCAI 2018, we have proposed a segmentation method based on simple image processing operators. Most of these operators come from the mathematical morphology framework. Driven by some prior knowledge on IVDs (basic information about their shape and the distance between them), and on their contrast in the different modalities, we were able to segment correctly almost every IVD. The most interesting feature of our method is to rely on the morphological structure called the Three of Shapes, which is another way to represent the image contents. This structure arranges all the connected components of an image obtained by thresholding into a tree, where each node represents a particular region. Such structure is actually powerful and versatile for pattern recognition tasks in medical imaging.

Keywords: Mathematical morphology · Tree of shapes

1 Introduction

Segmenting intervertebral discs (IVDs) is important to be able to measure automatically their degeneration. Indeed, there is a strong association between such degeneration and low back pain, which is one of the most prevalent health problems amongst population and, consequently, a leading cause of disability that affects work performances and well-being.

The recent trend in medical imaging segmentation is to use convolutional neural networks (CNN), which was not yet the case of the (rather) recent state-of-the-art methods such as [1,10,14,15]. Since many research groups would probably take advantage of the powerful—yet black-boxed–CNNs, we have decided to propose an alternative approach based on *mathematical morphology*. Section 2 explains the morphological tools used in our method, which is described in Sect. 3. The result we obtained on the data provided by the challenge "Automatic intervertebral disc localization and segmentation from 3D multi-modality

© Springer Nature Switzerland AG 2019
G. Zheng et al. (Eds.): CSI 2018, LNCS 11397, pp. 105–118, 2019.
https://doi.org/10.1007/978-3-030-13736-6_9

MR images (IVDM3Seg)"[1], that took place at the 21st International Conference on Medical Image Computing & Computer Assisted Intervention (MICCAI) 2018, are given in Sect. 4. As we advocate reproducible research, the code of the method presented here is available from: https://publications.lrde.epita.fr/carlinet.19.csi.

2   Theoretical Background

The method we propose falls into the framework of *mathematical morphology*. This section thus recalls the basic notions that are used in this paper. We will consider that an image, either a 2D digital image or a 3D digital volume, are represented by a function $f : X \to Y$, where X is a subset of $\mathbb{Z}^2$, resp. $\mathbb{Z}^3$, and where Y is a subset of $\mathbb{N}$, typically $[\![0, 255]\!]$ in the case of an 8-bit quantization.

2.1   Operators

An operator φ on images (i.e., taking an image as input and producing an image as output) is:

- increasing iff $f_1 \leq f_2 \Rightarrow \varphi(f_1) \leq \varphi(f_2)$,
- idempotent iff $\varphi \circ \varphi(f) = \varphi(f)$,
- extensive iff $\varphi(f) \geq f$,
- anti-extensive iff $\varphi(f) \leq f$.

In the writing of these properties, we implicitly consider that, for an operator φ, they apply whatever the considered functions. Furthermore, $\varphi \circ \varphi(f) = \varphi(f)$ means that $\forall x \in X$, we have $\varphi \circ \varphi(f)(x) = \varphi(f)(x)$. In the following, we will also use the classical operator *compact* notation, such as $\varphi \circ \varphi = \varphi$, meaning that such a property applies whatever the function. Last, we say that:

- the operators φ and ψ are dual iff $\varphi(f) = -\psi(-f)$,
- the operator φ is self-dual iff $\varphi(f) = -\varphi(-f)$.

2.2   Morphology with Structuring Elements

First let us recall the couple of fundamental operators of mathematical morphology. We call *structuring element*, a set B of vectors having the same discrete coordinate system than X. In the following, we will only consider structuring elements with the two following properties:

- centered, that is, $0 \in B$,
- and symmetrical, that is, $b \in B \Rightarrow -b \in B$.

---

[1] Site of the challenge: https://ivdm3seg.weebly.com/.

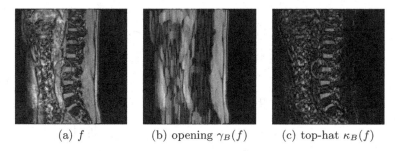

(a) f (b) opening $\gamma_B(f)$ (c) top-hat $\kappa_B(f)$

Fig. 1. Illustration of the white top-hat effect, with B being a vertical line of 15 pixels. (Color figure online)

The structuring element is a parameter for some morphological operators; its shape influences the filtering effect, while its size adjusts the filtering strength.

Given a structuring element B, the dilation δ and the erosion ε are operators on images, respectively defined by:

$$\forall x \in X, \ \delta_B(f)(x) = \max_{b \in B} f(x + b) \tag{1}$$

$$\varepsilon_B(f)(x) = \min_{b \in B} f(x + b). \tag{2}$$

These two operators are dual, so $\varepsilon_B(f) = -\delta_B(-f)$. The dilation is extensive (the resulting image is brighter than the input image), whereas the erosion is anti-extensive (the result is darker than the input).

From these two operators, we can define two idempotent operators, the closing (extensive) and the opening (anti-extensive), respectively by:

$$\phi_B = \varepsilon_B \circ \delta_B, \tag{3}$$

$$\gamma_B = \delta_B \circ \varepsilon_B, \tag{4}$$

which are dual: $\phi_B(f) = -\gamma_B(-f)$. If we consider that an image f is seen as a landscape, where $f(x)$ is the elevation—height of the landscape—at point x, the effect of the closing ϕ_B is to fill valleys, i.e., image parts surrounded (in the sense of B) by brighter pixels, whereas the opening γ_B has the opposite effect: remove mountains, i.e., image parts surrounded by darker pixels. The white top-hat operator is derived from the opening:

$$\kappa_B = \mathrm{id} - \gamma_B, \tag{5}$$

where "id" denotes the identity operator. Since we have $\kappa_B \leq \mathrm{id}$, the top-hat operator is anti-extensive: it removes some bright regions in images.

The behavior of the opening and top-hat operators are illustrated in Fig. 1. The IVD spaces appear as light parts in the original image f (Fig. 1(a)), surrounded *vertically* by some darker regions, that correspond to disks. Therefore the effect of an opening with a vertical structuring element is to remove the

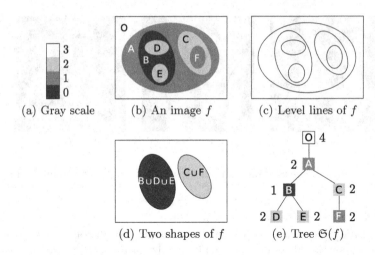

(a) Gray scale   (b) An image f (c) Level lines of f

(d) Two shapes of f (e) Tree $\mathfrak{S}(f)$

Fig. 2. Toy example of an image, its level lines, its shapes, and its tree of shapes.

bright IVD spaces, as it can be seen in Fig. 1(b). In this image, namely $\gamma_B(f)$, the part of the spine is exclusively dark.

The top-hat is the difference $\kappa_B(f) = f - \gamma_B(f)$, so the removed IVDs now reappear; this result is depicted in Fig. 1(c). When comparing the original image f with $\kappa_B(f)$, we can observe that most of the bright parts/objects of f have been filtered out, and, as a corollary, some IVD regions that were connected in f with some other anatomical parts are now de-connected in $\kappa_B(f)$; see for example the red circle in Fig. 1(a) and (c).

In the following, the top-hat operator will thus be used to "clean" the 3D volumes in different modalities, so that:

- many non-IVD objects are removed in the resulting volumes,
- and IVDs appear more clearly and are de-connected from other objects.

2.3   Tree of Shapes

Given a gray-level image $f : X \to Y$ and any scalar $\lambda \in Y$, the lower level sets are defined as:

$$[f < \lambda] = \{x \in X; f(x) < \lambda\}, \tag{6}$$

and the upper level sets as:

$$[f \geq \lambda] = \{x \in X; f(x) \geq \lambda\}. \tag{7}$$

We will now consider the connected components (obtained by the operator denoted by $\mathcal{CC}$) of these sets. Let us denote by Sat the cavity-fill-in operator[2]. In the following, we call *shape* the result of the cavity-fill-in operator applied to a connected component of a (lower or upper) level set. In the image f depicted in Fig. 2(b), we have for instance the lower level set $[f < 1] = \mathsf{B}$, and $\mathcal{CC}([f < 1]) = \{\mathsf{B}\}$. Note that B has two holes, namely D and E, so we have the shape $\mathrm{Sat}(\mathsf{B}) = \mathsf{B} \cup \mathsf{D} \cup \mathsf{E}$. An example of upper level set is $[f \geq 2]$, and $\mathcal{CC}([f \geq 2]) = \{\mathsf{C}, \mathsf{D}, \mathsf{E}\}$. C is a component of a level set, so $\mathrm{Sat}(\mathsf{C}) = \mathsf{C} \cup \mathsf{F}$ is a shape. Figure 2(d) depicts the two shapes $\mathrm{Sat}(\mathsf{B})$ and $\mathrm{Sat}(\mathsf{C})$.

The tree of shapes (ToS) of an image u is classically [13] defined by:

$$\mathfrak{S}(f) = \{\mathrm{Sat}(\Gamma); \ \Gamma \in \mathcal{CC}([f < \lambda]) \cup \mathcal{CC}([f \geq \lambda])\}_\lambda. \tag{8}$$

An image f and its tree of shapes $\mathfrak{S}(f)$ are depicted respectively in Fig. 2(b) and (e). An element of $\mathfrak{S}(f)$ is called a shape; it is a connected component of X with no cavity, and its boundary is a level line of f. Two shapes of f are displayed in Fig. 2(d). Every shape corresponds to a node of the tree; for instance, in Fig. 2(e) (right), the sub-tree rooted at node "B" corresponds to the shape $\mathsf{B} \cup \mathsf{D} \cup \mathsf{E}$. Keeping the level of every node—such as displayed in Fig. 2(e) (right)—allows to reconstruct the image from its tree. It is thus another way to represent the image contents.

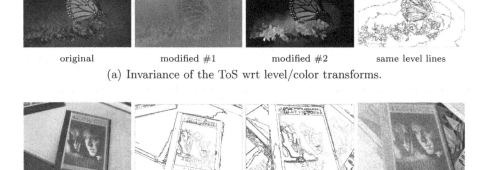

original   modified #1   modified #2   same level lines

(a) Invariance of the ToS wrt level/color transforms.

image #1   lines of #1   lines of #2   image #2

(b) Stability of level lines (taken from [19]).

Fig. 3. About properties of the tree of shapes and the level lines. (Color figure online)

It is worth mentioning that the tree of shapes has also been defined for multivariate data [5], that is, images whose pixel values are not scalars but vectors,

---

[2] Topological reminder: In 2D, the cavity-fill-in operator is also called hole filling; in 3D, a cavity is just like a bubble within a sphere (whereas a hole is like a tunnel going through a sphere).

such as it is the case for instance for color images, multi-modality medical images, and multi-band satellite images[3].

The tree of shapes of an image f is a morphological representation of f, which makes it easier to deal with the image contents [9]. For a "classical" image, there is about as many nodes in the tree than pixels in the image. Such a tree thus encodes a lot of shapes (connected components, i.e., regions) and their inclusion relationship. Despite one might think that such a structure should be complex and long to compute, and heavy to store in memory, this is actually not true. Indeed, storing [3] and computing [6,11,12] the tree of shapes can both be done *very efficiently*.

The tree of shapes is an operator satisfying two important major properties. First, we have:

$$\mathfrak{S}(-f) \;=\; \mathfrak{S}(f), \qquad\qquad (9)$$

meaning that this representation does not favor a particular contrast (light regions surrounded by darker ones, or the opposite). This property thus "contrasts" with the morphological operators presented in Sect. 2.3, where dual operators (such as δ and ε, or ϕ and γ) can be useful exactly because they rely on a particular kind of contrast: we choose one of the dual operators so that we process either brighter or darker parts of the images (remind Fig. 1 for instance). Conversely, the tree of shapes is a structure from which we can derive self-dual operators, that are, operators that process "the same way" light objects *and* dark objects. The second property is that, with any non-negative function ℓ acting over gray-levels (that is, a contrast change function), we have:

$$\mathfrak{S}(\ell \circ f) \;=\; \mathfrak{S}(f). \qquad\qquad (10)$$

This property implies that it is not the gray-level values of the pixels that matters, but only their ordering. Applying a gray-level change (or look-up table) such as $\ell = [0 \mapsto 0, 1 \mapsto 2, 2 \mapsto 4, 3 \mapsto 5]$ to the image in Fig. 2(b) does not change the structure of its tree of shapes: the ToS of the new image is the one of Fig. 2(e). As a direct consequence, the image processing operators that derive from the ToS structure apply the same way on low-contrasted images (or low-contrasted parts of images) than on better contrasted ones.

These properties are illustrated in Fig. 3. The image on the left in Fig. 3(a) has been modified to produce two new images. The modification #1 consists in contrast-change and contrast-inversion on the different color components; we have applied a function ℓ_i (such as in Eq. 10) on each ith component. The modification #2 is a *local* contrast change. In both cases, the original image and the modified ones have exactly the same set of level lines, depicted on the right. In Fig. 3(b), two images (on the left and on the right) share partially the same contents—a DVD jacket; yet the point of view, the lighting environment, and the quantity of noise are different. Despite these differences, the "meaningful"

---

[3] Such a multi-variate version of the tree of shapes is used in the illustrations of Figs. 3 and 4, but not in the segmentation method presented in this paper.

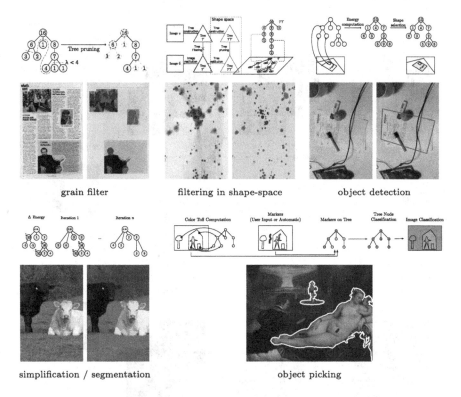

Fig. 4. Some applications of the ToS: grain filter [8], filtering in shape-space [17], object detection [16], simplification/segmentation [18], object picking [4]. (Color figure online)

level lines extracted from both images are very similar; the lines are depicted on the middle, the colors expressing the depth in their respective tree of shapes. In the grain filter example, depicted on the top-left part in Fig. 4, we can see that both bright and dark objects tiny are filtering out at the same time, thus illustrating the self-dual property, Eq. 9, of the ToS structure.

2.4 Some Applications of the Tree of Shapes

The tree of shapes is a versatile tool to perform image filtering [17], and a very relevant structure to perform some pattern recognition and computer vision tasks [2,7]. For illustration purpose, Fig. 4 shows that many applications can be derived from manipulating—or just using—the tree of shapes.

3 Method Description

In the IVDM3Seg challenge, for each patient we have four aligned high-resolution 3D volumes: in-phase, opposed-phase, fat and water images. We only use the three last modalities, abbreviated in the following `opp`, `fat`, and `wat` respectively.

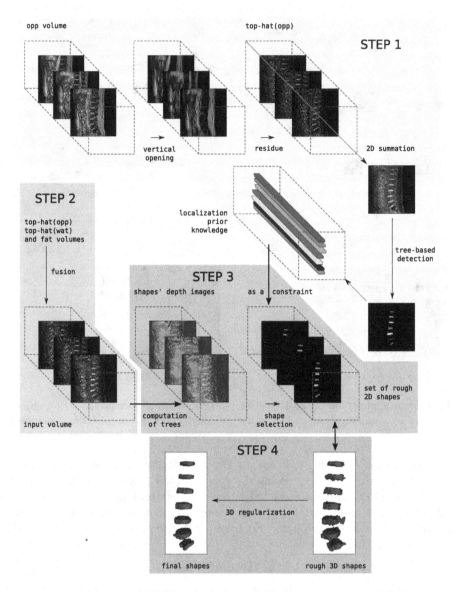

Fig. 5. Scheme of our method.

Our method has four main steps, illustrated in Fig. 5:

- Step 1: obtain some prior knowledge about IVDs localization, i.e., get a 2D region of interest (ROI) for each IVD;
- Step 2: prepare a 3D "input" volume from the volumes corresponding to the 3 modalities;
- Step 3: identify shapes that correspond to IVDs in the set of "input" slices, using the ROIs as localization constraints;

– Step 4: regularize the output in 3D.

These steps are described in the next four sections.

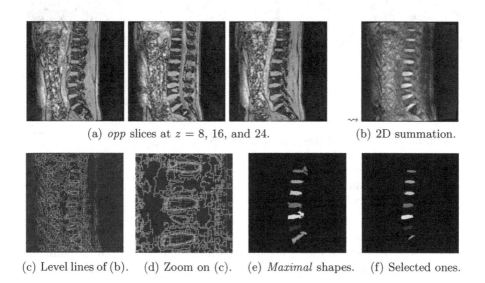

(a) *opp* slices at $z = 8$, 16, and 24.   (b) 2D summation.

(c) Level lines of (b).   (d) Zoom on (c).   (e) *Maximal* shapes.   (f) Selected ones.

Fig. 6. Step 1: obtaining localization prior knowledge.

3.1   Obtaining Prior Knowledge About IVDs Localization

The first step of the method aims at getting a gross estimation of the IVDs in 3D which will be refined later. At this stage, we do not need a precision at pixel level, only the bounding box of the IVDs.

Image Preprocessing. The method works with the *opp* volume only. In slices which reveal the IVDs the most, IVDs appear as bright oriented blobs which are at least 7-pixels high. Thus, for each slice, a top-hat (as described in Sect. 2.2) with a flat vertical structuring element of size 15×1 allows filtering out the background and highlights the IVDs. Then, the slices are summed up (similar to an Average Intensity Projection along the z-axis) to produce a consensus image. The projection serves as a Temporal Noise Reduction to reduce noisy structures that could have passed the top-hat filtering in some frames. Figure 6(b) shows the result of the preprocessing of a volume whose slices are shown in Fig. 6(a).

IVD Selection. The method computes the Tree of Shapes (ToS) on the preprocessed image. The latter enables a hierarchical representation of the inclusion of the hole-filled connected components of the image. The tree is then filtered by some prior-knowledge-based basic criteria:

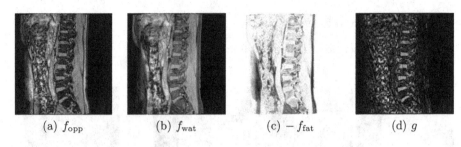

(a) f_{opp}　　　　(b) f_{wat}　　　　(c) $-f_{\mathrm{fat}}$　　　　(d) g

Fig. 7. Step 2: creation of a 3D volume from three different modalities.

- bounding box size and position of the shape
- position of the center of the shape
- orientation of the shape
- height of the shape
- average gray level of the shape.

Only about 20 maximal (i.e., not included in any other shape) shapes S_i are able to pass these requirements but have non-regular contours. To overcome this problem, we then look for the sub-shapes S_i^* the most compact (i.e., maximizing the ratio of the surface over the enclosing oriented rectangle surface) included in the maximal shapes S_i.

From this set of candidates, we then need to select only 7 of them—because exactly 7 IVDs are expected for the challenge. The candidates are sorted by decreasing average gray value (remind that IVDs appear very bright in the pre-processed image). The brightest shape serves as a reference and is augmented with shapes taken from S_i^* satisfying some relative positioning constraints:

- the y-distance between the shape center and the current bounding box is between 15 and 45 pixels
- the x-distance between the shape center and top/bottom selected shapes is below 15 pixels.

Figure 6(e) and (f) illustrate the 7 *maximal* and *regular* shapes retained by our shape selection algorithm. From these shapes, we extract the 7 Region of Interests (ROI) as the bounding boxes of the selected shapes. These ROIs and shape center will be used as markers in Step 3.

3.2 Preparing a 3D "input" Volume

The previously detected seeds are used to guide the search in the 2D slices. We are now going to work on an image combining the `opp`, `fat` and `wat` modalities, as IVDs contours may be spread among these images. To that aim, the top-hat filtering is used to enhance the contrast of IVDs. The combination of the 3 volumes is given by:

$$g = \kappa_B(f_{\mathrm{opp}}) + \kappa_B(f_{\mathrm{wat}}) - f_{\mathrm{wat}}, \tag{11}$$

and is illustrated in Fig. 7.

3.3   Identifying Shapes of IVDs in 2D Slices

This step is very similar to the *IDV Selection* process of Step 2 described in Sect. 3.1. A ToS is computed on each slice of the 3D input volume. In each ROI of the IVDs localized previously, we look for the best *regular* shape passing some basic geometric criteria (min/max size, bounding box, minimum intensity...). Note that for an IVD ROI, there may not exist such shape, as some IVDs might not be visible in some slices.

3.4   3D Regularization

Z-axis Regularization: In some slices, when no shape can be found for a given IVD, it may be normal but also might be a missed detection. If a pixel (x, y) is labeled at $z = k - 1$ and $z = k + 1$, but not at slice $z = k$, it is likely a miss-detection. As a consequence, the regularization applies:

$$f(z, x, y) = f(z, x, y) \vee (f(z - 1, x, y) \wedge f(z + 1, x, y))$$

3D Shape Regularization: In each 2D slice, shapes are quite *regular* because of the shape selection algorithm that favors regular contours. On the contrary, back in 3D, the concatenation of 2D results has no 3D coherence. To tackle this problem, a structural opening followed by a structural closing with a small 3D ball allows to remove contour irregularities.

Isolated Pixels Removal: While the *z-axis regularization* tackles the missed-detection problem, false-detections may appear due to some natural noise (especially at the beginning and the end of the sequence). These shapes are generally disconnected in 3D from the real IVDs. Thus, as a final step, we perform a 3D connected component labeling and only retain the 7 largest ones.

Step 4 in Fig. 5 illustrates the 3D regularization of the shapes performed by our method.

	Dice
mean	0.881
sd	0.025
min	0.852
max	0.927

(a) On the training set.

	IVDs						
	1	2	3	4	5	6	7
1	0.784	—	—	0.858	0.589	0.850	0.659
2	0.899	0.416	—	0.916	0.902	0.892	0.706
3	0.742	—	—	0.787	0.815	0.732	0.601
4	0.813	0.908	0.910	0.837	0.832	0.793	0.763
5	—	0.805	0.911	0.879	0.864	0.875	0.659
6	—	0.723	0.902	0.883	0.882	0.857	0.635
7	0.839	0.902	0.900	0.888	0.872	0.839	0.784
8	0.847	0.896	0.892	0.897	0.890	0.863	—
mean	0.821	0.775	0.903	0.868	0.831	0.838	0.687

(b) Dice values on the 8 cases of the test set.

Fig. 8. Quantitative results on the challenge data sets.

4   Results

First we have run our method on the 16 cases of the challenge training set. We can observe in Fig. 8(a) that the average Dice value of **0.881** is good, with a very low standard deviation. On the 8 cases of the test set, the different rows in Fig. 8(b), we miss some IVDs (which is symbolized by "—" in the table). Since we do not have access to the data of the test set, we cannot figure out what makes our method fail for these few IVDs. Yet, for the ones we segment, the Dice values are satisfactory, with an overall average Dice of **0.816**. Last, some qualitative results, compared to the reference images provided by the challenge organizers, are depicted in Fig. 9.

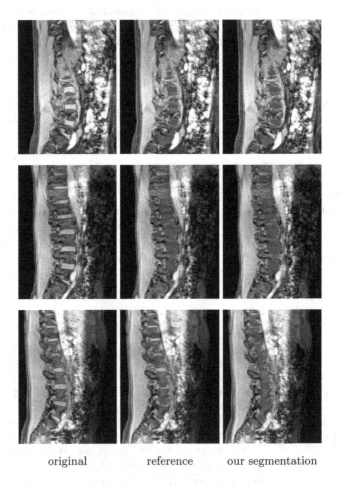

original   reference   our segmentation

Fig. 9. Some qualitative results on selected slices, respectively taken from training samples #6 (top), #14 (middle), and #16 (bottom).

5 Conclusion

We have presented a mathematical morpholology-based of the IVD segmentation problem. This method which is a machine-learning free, only relies on a chain of some simple morphological processing blocks. Despite being a learning-free approach, we have shown that it is able to compete with new CNN-based methods (but still perform worst when looking at the metrics only). On the other hand, the strength of our method lies in its speed. Only few seconds are required to process a whole volume with a single-threaded desktop processor, where CNN-based methods would be several order of magnitude slower. Yet, our implementation does not take benefit neither from a straightforward parallelization of the 2D slices processing, nor from parallel implementations of the tree of shapes [6,11].

References

1. Ben Ayed, I., Punithakumar, K., Garvin, G., Romano, W., Li, S.: Graph cuts with invariant object-interaction priors: application to intervertebral disc segmentation. In: Székely, G., Hahn, H.K. (eds.) IPMI 2011. LNCS, vol. 6801, pp. 221–232. Springer, Heidelberg (2011). https://doi.org/10.1007/978-3-642-22092-0_19

2. Cao, F., Lisani, J.L., Morel, J.M., Musé, P., Sur, F.: A Theory of Shape Identification. LNM, vol. 1948. Springer, Heidelberg (2008). https://doi.org/10.1007/978-3-540-68481-7

3. Carlinet, E., Géraud, T.: A comparative review of component tree computation algorithms. IEEE Trans. Image Process. **23**(9), 3885–3895 (2014)

4. Carlinet, E., Géraud, T.: Morphological object picking based on the color tree of shapes. In: Proceedings of the 5th International Conference on Image Processing Theory, Tools and Applications (IPTA), Orléans, France, pp. 125–130, November 2015

5. Carlinet, E., Géraud, T.: MToS: a tree of shapes for multivariate images. IEEE Trans. Image Process. **24**(12), 5330–5342 (2015)

6. Carlinet, E., Géraud, T., Crozet, S.: The tree of shapes turned into a max-tree: a simple and efficient linear algorithm. In: Proceedings of the 24th IEEE International Conference on Image Processing (ICIP), Athens, Greece, pp. 1488–1492, October 2018

7. Caselles, V., Coll, B., Morel, J.M.: Topographic maps and local contrast changes in natural images. Int. J. Comput. Vis. **33**(1), 5–27 (1999)

8. Caselles, V., Monasse, P.: Grain filters. J. Math. Imaging Vis. **17**(3), 249–270 (2002)

9. Caselles, V., Monasse, P.: Geometric Description of Images as Topographic Maps. LNM, vol. 1984. Springer, Heidelberg (2009). https://doi.org/10.1007/978-3-642-04611-7

10. Chen, C., et al.: Localization and segmentation of 3D intervertebral discs in MR images by data driven estimation. IEEE Trans. Med. Imaging **34**(8), 1719–1729 (2015)

11. Crozet, S., Géraud, T.: A first parallel algorithm to compute the morphological tree of shapes of nD images. In: Proceedings of the 21st IEEE International Conference on Image Processing (ICIP), Paris, France, pp. 2933–2937 (2014)

12. Géraud, T., Carlinet, E., Crozet, S., Najman, L.: A quasi-linear algorithm to compute the tree of shapes of nD images. In: Hendriks, C.L.L., Borgefors, G., Strand, R. (eds.) ISMM 2013. LNCS, vol. 7883, pp. 98–110. Springer, Heidelberg (2013). https://doi.org/10.1007/978-3-642-38294-9_9

13. Monasse, P., Guichard, F.: Fast computation of a contrast-invariant image representation. IEEE Trans. Image Process. **9**(5), 860–872 (2000)

14. Neubert, A., Fripp, J., Engstrom, C., Walker, D., Weber, M.: Three-dimensional morphological and signal intensity features for detection of intervertebral disc degeneration from magnetic resonance images. J. Am. Med. Inform. Assoc. **20**(6), 1082–1090 (2013)

15. Stern, D., Likar, B., Pernus, F., Vrtovec, T.: Automated detection of spinal centrelines, vertebral bodies and intervertebral discs in CT and MR images of lumbar spine. Phys. Med. Biol. **55**(1), 247–264 (2010)

16. Xu, Y., Carlinet, E., Géraud, T., Najman, L.: Hierarchical segmentation using tree-based shape spaces. IEEE Trans. Pattern Anal. Mach. Intell. **39**(3), 457–469 (2017)

17. Xu, Y., Géraud, T., Najman, L.: Connected filtering on tree-based shape-spaces. IEEE Trans. Pattern Anal. Mach. Intell. **38**(6), 1126–1140 (2016)

18. Xu, Y., Géraud, T., Najman, L.: Hierarchical image simplification and segmentation based on Mumford-Shah-salient level line selection. Pattern Recogn. Lett. **83**(3), 278–286 (2016)

19. Xu, Y., Monasse, P., Géraud, T., Najman, L.: Tree-based morse regions: a topological approach to local feature detection. IEEE Trans. Image Process. **23**(12), 5612–5625 (2014)

Deep Learning Framework for Fully Automated Intervertebral Disc Localization and Segmentation from Multi-modality MR Images

Yunhe Gao[1,2(✉)]

[1] Department of Electronic Engineering, The Chinese University of Hong Kong,
Shatin N.T., Hong Kong
yhgao@link.cuhk.edu.hk
[2] SenseTime Group, Beijing, China

Abstract. Intervertebral discs are joints that lie between vertebrae in the spinal column, which absorb shock between vertebrae during activities. There is a strong correlation between lower back pain and degeneration of intervertebral discs, which may have a great impact on peoples normal life. The precise segmentation of the intervertebral disc is of great significance for the diagnosis of disc degeneration. Currently clinical practice usually manually annotates the volumetric data, which is time-consuming, tedious, needs a lot of expertise and lacks of reproducibility. In this challenge, we developed a fully automated framework that can accurately segment and locate seven intervertebral discs. First, we delicately designed a powerful segmentation network which is a 2D fully convolutional neural network with densely connected atrous spatial pyramid pooling to capture and fuse multi-scale context information. Then we used a localization network and a robust post-process scheme to distinguish different IVD instance. Further more, we proposed a novel training strategy that can make the segmentation network focus on the spine region. The effectiveness of our algorithm is proven in the challenge, we achieved the mean segmentation Dice coefficient of 90.58% and a mean localization error of 0.78 mm.

Keywords: IVD localization · IVD segmentation · Deep learning

1 Introduction

The intervertebral disc is a fibrocartilage disc that connects adjacent vertebrae so that the spine can move within a certain angle. The IVDs have the nature of toughness and elasticity, and can be deformed under pressure, so that the force applied on the IVDs can be evenly distributed into all directions, and ensure the entire surface of vertebral is subjected to the same pressure. IVDs are also the main structure for absorbing shock. When the human body jumps, falls from

© Springer Nature Switzerland AG 2019
G. Zheng et al. (Eds.): CSI 2018, LNCS 11397, pp. 119–129, 2019.
https://doi.org/10.1007/978-3-030-13736-6_10

a high place, and performs other vertical movements, or when the shoulders, back, and waist suddenly load heavy objects, the IVDs can buffer the force by conduction and self-deformation, hence plays the role of protecting the spinal cord and vital organs in the body.

However, with age, excessive activity or overload, it may lead to degeneration of the intervertebral disc, causing lower back pain, numbness of lower limb, nerve injury or even loss of movement, which will seriously affect work ability and life quality. Clinically, medical image analysis is usually the best non-invasive diagnostic method. In order to obtain quantitative parameters, doctors usually manually annotate the IVDs. However, for 3D images, this method is usually tedious, time-consuming, needs a lot of expertise and lack of reproducibility. Therefore, a fully automatic localization and segmentation algorithm of the intervertebral disc can offer visualized 3D reconstructed image and also provide quantitative parameters, which can greatly improve the speed as well as the quality of the diagnosis.

As magnetic resonance imaging has the properties of excellent sensitivity to soft tissue and no radiation, it is widely considered to be the best modality for disc disease diagnosis. Further more, the Dixon method can generate fat only and water only images by combining the in-phase and opposed-phase signal. Making full use of the image information from different modalities can improve the accuracy of the segmentation algorithm. The four modality Dixon sequences are showed in Fig. 1.

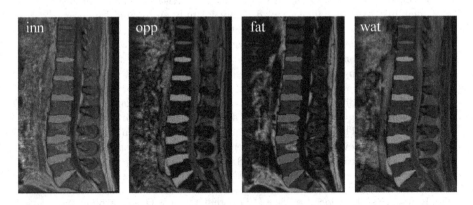

Fig. 1. Examples of multi-modality Dixon sequence, including in-phase, opposed-phase, fat and water from left to right. Each modality has different contrasts for specific components, making full use of multi-modality information can result in better contour segmentation. It should be noted that there are more than seven IVDs in the MR images, but only the lumber IVDs are our objective.

The task of this challenge has two parts, the localization and segmentation of intervertebral disc. The objective of segmentation is to obtain the binary mask of each IVD, i.e. each voxel in the image is classified into the disc category or non-disc category. The objective of localization is to obtain the coordinates of the centroid of each disc, which is calculated by the morphological center of each IVD mask. The segmentation algorithm affects both segmentation accuracy and localization accuracy, therefore a good segmentation algorithm is a prerequisite.

1.1 Related Work

In early studies, researchers typically used hand-crafted features [4,14] based on image intensity or texture features for IVD localization and segmentation. Graph-based methods are commonly used in the segmentation of vertebrae and discs. For example normalized cut [2] and graph cut algorithm [1] were used for IVDs segmentation in spine MR images. And graphical models [5,12] were used for IVD localization.

As learning-based approaches gain more and more attention in the medical image analysis field, several marginal spacing learning [9] and regression-based methods [3] are proposed for localize IVDs and segment IVDs. However, those methods were limited by the representation capability of the hand-crafted features.

Recently, deep learning methods have revolutionized medical image analysis and computer vision field with its remarkable feature representation capability. For example, Ronneberger et al. [13] proposed U-net for cell segmentation from 2D images and Dou et al. [6] proposed 3D convolutional neural network for 3D liver cancer segmentation. Deep learning methods also improve the performance of IVD localization and segmentation to a brand new level. For example, Li et al. [10] proposed a 3D multi-scale FCN with random modality dropout scheme to better utilize multi-modality information and achieved decent accuracy for IVD localization and segmentation.

1.2 Contribution

We propose a strong and robust deep learning framework for IVDs localization and segmentation from multi-modality MR images. The evaluation results from *MICCAI 2018 Automatic Intervertebral Disc Localization and Segmentation from 3D Multi-modality MR Images* demonstrated the effectiveness of our proposed framework. Our main contributions can be summarized as follows:

- We delicately design a 2D fully convolutional network, which only performs downsampling for 2 times, and use densely connected atrous spatial pyramid pooling to capture multi-scale features as well as ensure large enough receptive field. The network consists of three separate pathways for different spatial resolution features, which makes the training of encoder more effective. Further more, a Squeeze-and-Excitation module are used for channel-wise attention. This network is a strong backbone that can be generalized to other medical image segmentation tasks.

- We designed a 3D V-Net based localization network with a robust post-process scheme to classify the seven lumber disc into seven category and distinguish them from other thoracic discs, which makes the whole framework to be fully automated.
- We proposed a novel and intuitive training strategy that can make the segmentation network focus on the spine region while ignore the interference from large and complex backgrounds.
- Our method was evaluated on MICCAI 2018 IVDM3Seg dataset which consists of 16 sets of 3D multi-modality MR images from 8 subjects, and demonstrated superior performance.

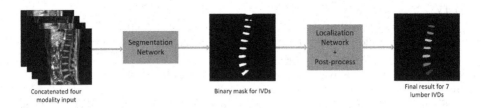

Fig. 2. The pipeline of proposed framework for IVD localization and segmentation. The segmentation first perform binary segmentation to classify each voxel into disc and non-disc region. The localization network and post-process treat each disc instance as a categories and assign label from 1–7 from bottom to top.

2   Methodology

The pipeline of our framework for IVD localization and segmentation are illustrated in Fig. 2. Our localization and segmentation framework mainly consists of two parts: the segmentation network, the localization network and the post-process scheme. The objective of segmentation is to output the binary masks of each IVD, however, because of the similarity between thoracic discs and lumber discs, the segmentation network will predict more than 7 IVD masks, though only 7 lumber discs have annotation. To obtain the final result and achieve the purpose of fully automation, we designed a V-Net based localization network which treats each IVD as an instance, i.e. performs 7 class segmentation, and then used a post-processing method to increase the robustness of the localization network.

2.1   Segmentation Network

In recent years, convolutional neural networks have revolutionized the field of computer vision and medical image analysis. 2D CNNs based methods have made great progress on medical images compared to traditional methods. Recently, 3D CNNs [6,11] are explored as they can capture volumetric contextual information

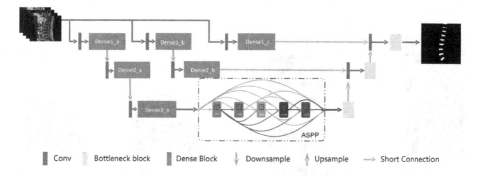

Fig. 3. The proposed 2D fully convolutional segmentation network, it takes the 4-channel concatenated multi-modality image as input, and outputs the binary mask of IVDs.

and have better representation capability. However, 3D CNNs essentially have a disadvantage compared to 2D CNNs, they have a greater demand for data, as 3D CNNs treat a volumetric image as a single sample while 2D CNNs treat each slice as a single sample. There are only 16 samples in the training set, therefore, we think the 2D network is more suitable for this task.

U-net [13] is one of the most successful 2D convolutional neural networks in medical image analysis, many previous deep learning methods are modified based on it. U-net has a symmetric Encoder-Decoder structure, the encoder encodes multi-scale information into feature maps by four downsamplings. The decoder then reconstruct spatial resolution from high-level feature maps by upsampling or deconvolution, while high-resolution features are also concatenated by short connection from encoder to assist reconstruction. However, this structure has three inherent defect for semantic segmentation. First, too many times of downsampling leads to the loss of detail information, although the high-resolution feature maps are used in the reconstruction process, but this low-level feature concatenate and feature fusion can only slightly alleviate the problem. Second, UNet captures multi-scale features by downsapling, which results in capturing only fixed and limited scales of features, making it difficult to represent complex and variable anatomical structures. Third, during the gradient back propagation in the training phase, the encoder will receive two gradient signals from different resolutions, one is the low resolution gradient signal from below, and the other is the same resolution gradient signal from the shortcut connection. It cannot be guaranteed that the two path have the same magnitude of gradient signal because the number of convolution layers on different paths is quite different. The mixing of these two signals in the training process will affect the effectiveness of the encoder training.

To solve the problems mentioned above, we elaborately design our segmentation network, see in Fig. 3. We use a strong backbone network, which is based on DenseNet [8] and uses Squeeze-and-Excitation module [7] as channel-wise attention. For the first problem, reduce the number of downsampling is a intu-

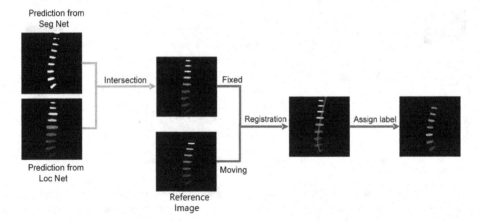

Fig. 4. The pipeline of localization network and the post-process scheme. (Color figure online)

itive solution. In the trade-off between the GPU memory usage and segmentation accuracy, our network only perform two downsamplings, it can effectively reduce the information loss, and improve the segmentation accuracy of the detailed edge region of discs. However, such structure has a disadvantage that the network can only fuse less scales of features, moreover, the receptive field of convolution kernel become smaller, which makes it difficult to capture more global and high-level features. Therefore, we further use densely connected dilated convolution to solve this problem, or use another name, densely connected atrous spatial pyramid pooling (ASPP). Compared with the serial connected or parallel connected [15] counterpart, densely connected ASPP combines arbitrary scales of features, which can be adjusted by dilation rate, and better feature reuse. In our model, we use the dilation rate of 3, 6, 12, 18 and 24. For the third problem, inspired by some works on multi-task learning, we design three separate paths to handle different resolution signal, i.e. treat each resolution signal path as a single task. This approach can train each path more effectively without interfering with each other.

2.2 Localization Network and Post-process

Although the segmentation network is trained only with 7 lumbar discs annotation, the network predicts more than 7 IVDs because of the similar anatomy pattern of thoracic disc and the lumbar disc. We design a localization network and a post-process scheme to handle the output of the segmentation network, and fully automatically get the target mask of 7 lumbar discs. The structure is shown in Fig. 4. The localization network has a V-Net structure, which is a 3D fully convolutional neural network with residual connection. The ground truth annotation of the localization network is obtained by marking the mask of the 7 IVDs in the original annotation from 1 to 7 from bottom to top, that is, the localization network output 8 channels score map, including seven IVDs and one background.

Then the prediction from localization network and prediction from segmentation network are intersected together. Due to the similar appearance of the IVDs, the predicted mask from localization network in the often have misclassified areas in the upper part of images, but the segmentation of the bottom disc is always right. We then use a reference image from training set as moving image to be registered to the predicted mask, and fit the centerline of spine from the centroid of each disc in the registered mask, i.e. the red line shown in Fig. 4. At last, we calculate the connected area of the predicted mask. Only the connected area that intersects with the fitted centerline of the spine is retained. The other connected regions are set as background. Then, the reserved connected region is assigned with label from 1 to 7 from bottom to top.

This localization and post-processing strategy can greatly improve the robustness of the framework, even if there are some misclassified outliers in the segmentation network, it will not affect the identify of IVDs.

2.3 Training Strategy

To further improve the performance of the segmentation network, we made a natural assumption.

Assumption. Only the spine part of the entire input image is useful for IVD segmentation, while region outside the spine only acts as a useless background, which will reduce the accuracy of the segmentation performance.

We first train a UNet to predict the spine area, where the label was generated by calculating the convex hull of the annotation of discs after several dilation operations. When training the segmentation network, the predicted mask from the UNet was used, and we ignore the loss outside the spine region. In the inference phase, the spine region is also predicted, and all the region outside the spine is set as background in the output of segmentation network.

2.4 Loss Function

When training segmentation network, focal loss was used for better focus on hard samples, i.e. the boundary region of IVDs, and the formula is as follow:

$$L(p) = -\alpha(1 - p)^{\gamma} log(p), \tag{1}$$

Since the use of focal loss may cause instability problems when training, we first train several epochs using cross entropy loss, then use focal loss.

3 Experiments

3.1 Dataset and Data Augmentation

We evaluated our proposed method on the dataset from MICCAI 2018 IVDM3Seg Challenge using both cross validation on the training data and independent test data on the on-site challenge, where training data consists of 16 sets of 3D multi-modality MR images from 8 subjects, and test data consists of 8 sets of 3D multi-modality MR images from 4 subjects. Each subject was scanned with a 1.5-Tesla MRI scanner of Siemens using Dixon protocol. The voxel spacing of each image is $2\,mm \times 1.25\,mm \times 1.25\,mm$. For the data augmentation, we use 3D deformation, random scale, random noise, and random crop.

3.2   Evaluation Metrics

Dice overlap coefficient measures the percentage of correctly segmented voxels. Dice is computed by

$$Dice(A, B) = \frac{2\,|\,A \cap B\,|}{|\,A\,| + |\,B\,|} \times 100\%, \tag{2}$$

where A is the sets of foreground voxels in the ground-truth data and B is the corresponding sets of foreground voxels in the segmentation result, respectively.

Average absolute distance (ASD) is a metric measures the average absolute distance from the ground truth disc surface and the segmented surface. Smaller average absolute distance means better segmentation accuracy.

Localization distance R is computed by

$$R = \sqrt{(\Delta x)^2 + (\Delta y)^2 + (\Delta z)^2}, \tag{3}$$

where Δx, Δy, Δz is the absolute difference between the identified IVD center and the ground truth IVD center calculated from the ground truth segmentation in X, Y and Z axis. Smaller localization distance means better segmentation accuracy.

3.3   Results of MICCAI 2018 and Training Set Cross Validation

The evaluation result of the on-site challenge of MICCAI 2018 IVDM3Seg are listed in Tables 1, 2 and 3. Our method demonstrated good performance and strong robustness. Since the test data are not available to us, the segmentation result are visualized using training set cross validation, see in Fig. 5.

Table 1. Dice overlap coefficient of independent test set in on-site challenge.

Dice	Disc_01	Disc_02	Disc_03	Disc_04	Disc_05	Disc_06	Disc_07
Test_01	0.888	0.904	0.927	0.911	0.896	0.890	0.868
Test_02	0.908	0.934	0.940	0.944	0.930	0.923	0.925
Test_03	0.894	0.896	0.900	0.866	0.896	0.818	0.884
Test_04	0.918	0.938	0.938	0.913	0.909	0.885	0.925
Test_05	0.897	0.911	0.917	0.918	0.869	0.896	0.926
Test_06	0.865	0.914	0.929	0.910	0.898	0.898	0.892
Test_07	0.904	0.931	0.931	0.914	0.904	0.887	0.863
Test_08	0.904	0.928	0.922	0.923	0.910	0.907	0.889

Table 2. Average absolute distance of independent test set in on-site challenge.

ASD(mm)	Disc_01	Disc_02	Disc_03	Disc_04	Disc_05	Disc_06	Disc_07
Test_01	0.73	0.67	0.49	0.58	0.63	0.61	0.68
Test_02	0.54	0.47	0.44	0.37	0.44	0.41	0.41
Test_03	0.72	0.82	0.74	0.87	0.57	0.90	0.54
Test_04	0.55	0.48	0.42	0.50	0.48	0.51	0.29
Test_05	0.58	0.70	0.69	0.61	0.97	0.68	0.37
Test_06	0.85	0.66	0.57	0.75	0.78	0.69	0.55
Test_07	0.64	0.53	0.52	0.64	0.62	0.65	0.65
Test_08	0.72	0.63	0.63	0.68	0.62	0.57	0.58

Table 3. Average absolute distance of independent test set in on-site challenge.

Localization(mm)	Disc_01	Disc_02	Disc_03	Disc_04	Disc_05	Disc_06	Disc_07
Test_01	0.44	1.42	0.53	0.78	1.37	0.98	1.08
Test_02	0.38	0.73	0.27	0.47	0.73	0.41	0.18
Test_03	0.64	0.33	1.36	2.11	0.95	1.27	0.46
Test_04	0.83	0.53	0.63	1.35	0.50	1.20	0.08
Test_05	0.80	0.34	0.13	1.04	0.93	1.04	0.49
Test_06	1.23	0.47	0.43	0.12	0.64	1.09	0.66
Test_07	0.60	1.12	0.98	1.21	1.17	0.63	1.07
Test_08	0.28	1.30	0.77	0.92	1.03	0.35	0.60

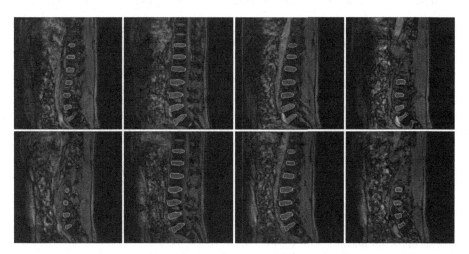

Fig. 5. Visualization of one subject in training set cross validation, the green line is the prediction of our approach, read line is ground truth and yellow line is the intersection. These images are from subject 3, the images in the first row is obtained in the first phase, while the second row is obtained in the second phase. (Color figure online)

4 Conclusion

In this paper, we present our novel and robust IVD segmentation and localization framework from multi-modality MR images, which achieve state-of-the-art performance. The delicately designed segmentation network can preserve the detailed information as much as possible by reducing the number of downsamplings, and at the same time, using densely connected atrous spatial pyramid pooling to capture and fuse multi-scale information as well as reserve large enough receptive field, which can greatly enhance the feature representation ability of the network. We also design three separate paths to handle different resolution signal to train each path more effectively. A new training strategy is also proposed to prevent the segmentation network from interfered by the large complex background. Furthermore, we propose a localization network with robust post-process scheme to distinguish thoracic discs and lumber discs. The result of MICCAI 2018 challenge on IVD localization and segmentation demonstrated the effectiveness of our proposed method.

References

1. Ben Ayed, I., Punithakumar, K., Garvin, G., Romano, W., Li, S.: Graph cuts with invariant object-interaction priors: application to intervertebral disc segmentation. In: Székely, G., Hahn, H.K. (eds.) IPMI 2011. LNCS, vol. 6801, pp. 221–232. Springer, Heidelberg (2011). https://doi.org/10.1007/978-3-642-22092-0_19
2. Carballido-Gamio, J., Belongie, S.J., Majumdar, S.: Normalized cuts in 3-D for spinal mri segmentation. IEEE Trans. Med. Imaging **23**(1), 36–44 (2004)
3. Chen, C., et al.: Localization and segmentation of 3D intervertebral discs in mr images by data driven estimation. IEEE Trans. Med. Imaging **34**(8), 1719–1729 (2015)
4. Chevrefils, C., Cheriet, F., Aubin, C.É., Grimard, G.: Texture analysis for automatic segmentation of intervertebral disks of scoliotic spines from mr images. IEEE Trans. Inf. Technol. Biomed. **13**(4), 608–620 (2009)
5. Corso, J.J., Alomari, R.S., Chaudhary, V.: Lumbar disc localization and labeling with a probabilistic model on both pixel and object features. In: Metaxas, D., Axel, L., Fichtinger, G., Székely, G. (eds.) MICCAI 2008. LNCS, vol. 5241, pp. 202–210. Springer, Heidelberg (2008). https://doi.org/10.1007/978-3-540-85988-8_25
6. Dou, Q., Chen, H., Jin, Y., Yu, L., Qin, J., Heng, P.-A.: 3D deeply supervised network for automatic liver segmentation from CT volumes. In: Ourselin, S., Joskowicz, L., Sabuncu, M.R., Unal, G., Wells, W. (eds.) MICCAI 2016. LNCS, vol. 9901, pp. 149–157. Springer, Cham (2016). https://doi.org/10.1007/978-3-319-46723-8_18
7. Hu, J., Shen, L., Sun, G.: Squeeze-and-excitation networks. arXiv preprint arXiv:1709.01507 (2017)
8. Huang, G., Liu, Z., Van Der Maaten, L., Weinberger, K.Q.: Densely connected convolutional networks. In: CVPR, vol. 1, p. 3 (2017)
9. Kelm, B.M., et al.: Spine detection in CT and MR using iterated marginal space learning. Med. Image Anal. **17**(8), 1283–1292 (2013)
10. Li, X., et al.: 3D multi-scale FCN with random modality voxel dropout learning for intervertebral disc localization and segmentation from multi-modality MR images. Med. Image Anal. **45**, 41–54 (2018)

11. Milletari, F., Navab, N., Ahmadi, S.A.: V-net: fully convolutional neural networks for volumetric medical image segmentation. In: 2016 Fourth International Conference on 3D Vision (3DV), pp. 565–571. IEEE (2016)
12. Raja'S, A., Corso, J.J., Chaudhary, V.: Labeling of lumbar discs using both pixel- and object-level features with a two-level probabilistic model. IEEE Trans. Med. Imaging **30**(1), 1–10 (2011)
13. Ronneberger, O., Fischer, P., Brox, T.: U-Net: convolutional networks for biomedical image segmentation. In: Navab, N., Hornegger, J., Wells, W.M., Frangi, A.F. (eds.) MICCAI 2015. LNCS, vol. 9351, pp. 234–241. Springer, Cham (2015). https://doi.org/10.1007/978-3-319-24574-4_28
14. Schmidt, S., et al.: Spine detection and labeling using a parts-based graphical model. In: Karssemeijer, N., Lelieveldt, B. (eds.) IPMI 2007. LNCS, vol. 4584, pp. 122–133. Springer, Heidelberg (2007). https://doi.org/10.1007/978-3-540-73273-0_11
15. Zhao, H., Shi, J., Qi, X., Wang, X., Jia, J.: Pyramid scene parsing network. In: IEEE Conference on Computer Vision and Pattern Recognition (CVPR), pp. 2881–2890 (2017)

IVD-Net: Intervertebral Disc Localization and Segmentation in MRI with a Multi-modal UNet

Jose Dolz[(✉)], Christian Desrosiers, and Ismail Ben Ayed

ETS Montreal, Montreal, Canada
{jose.dolz,christian.desrosiers,ismail.benayed}@etsmtl.ca

Accurate localization and segmentation of intervertebral disc (IVD) is crucial for the assessment of spine disease diagnosis. Despite the technological advances in medical imaging, IVD localization and segmentation are still manually performed, which is time-consuming and prone to errors. If, in addition, multi-modal imaging is considered, the burden imposed on disease assessments increases substantially. In this paper, we propose an architecture for IVD localization and segmentation in multi-modal magnetic resonance images (MRI), which extends the well-known UNet. Compared to single images, multi-modal data brings complementary information, contributing to better data representation and discriminative power. Our contributions are three-fold. First, how to effectively integrate and fully leverage multi-modal data remains almost unexplored. In this work, each MRI modality is processed in a different path to better exploit their unique information. Second, inspired by HyperDenseNet [11], the network is densely-connected both within each path and across different paths, granting the model the freedom to learn *where* and *how* the different modalities should be processed and combined. Third, we improved standard U-Net modules by extending inception modules [22] with two convolutional blocks with dilated convolutions of different scale, which helps handling multi-scale context. We report experiments over the data set of the public MICCAI 2018 Challenge on Automatic Intervertebral Disc Localization and Segmentation, with 13 multi-modal MRI images used for training and 3 for validation. We trained IVD-Net on an NVidia TITAN XP GPU with 16 GBs RAM, using ADAM as optimizer and a learning rate of 1×10^{-5} during 200 epochs. Training took about 5 h, and segmentation of a whole volume about 2–3 s, on average. Several baselines, with different multi-modal fusion strategies, were used to demonstrate the effectiveness of the proposed architecture.

1   Introduction

Intervertebral disc (IVD) degeneration [1] is one of the main causes for chronic low back pain (LBP), which has become a major public health problem in our society and a leading cause of function incapacity [24]. Magnetic resonance imaging (MRI) is the preferred modality to evaluate lumbar degenerative disc disease because it offers a good soft tissue contrast without ionizing radiation [12].

© Springer Nature Switzerland AG 2019
G. Zheng et al. (Eds.): CSI 2018, LNCS 11397, pp. 130–143, 2019.
https://doi.org/10.1007/978-3-030-13736-6_11

Advances in multi-modal MRI have increased the quality of diagnosis, treatment and follow-up in many diseases. However this comes at the cost of an increased amount of data, imposing a burden on disease assessments. Visual inspections of such an enormous amount of medical images are prohibitively time-consuming, prone to errors and unsuitable for large-scale studies. Developing robust methods for automatic IVD localization and segmentation from multi-modal MRI is thus essential for the diagnosis and treatment of spine pathologies. Having such methods could also reduce the manual work required by clinicians, and provide a faster and more consistent diagnosis.

Over the years, various semi-automated and automated techniques have been proposed for IVD localization and segmentation [2,4]. Recently, deep convolutional neural networks (CNNs) have shown outstanding performance for this task, outperforming previous segmentation approaches [5,14,16,27,31]. For example, Ji et al. [14] proposed a standard CNN for IVD segmentation, where the inference was performed pixel-wise by extracting a patch around each pixel. In addition, the authors evaluated different patch strategies, such as 2D or 2.5D patches, as well as the impact of vicinity size. More recently, a deeply supervised multi-scale fully CNN was proposed in [27] for the segmentation of IVDs in MR-T2 weighted images. An interesting feature of this work is its use of multi-scale deep supervision in the architecture, which alleviates the risk of vanishing gradient during training. Despite achieving satisfactory results, these works have mostly focused on single-modality scenarios.

Integrating multi-modal images in deep learning segmentation methods has also gained growing attention recently. Multi-modal segmentation in CNNs is typically addressed with an *early fusion* strategy, where multiple modalities are merged from the original input space of low-level features [10,15,18,23,29] (See Fig. 1, *left*). By concatenating image modalities at the input of the network, we explicitly assume that the relation between different modalities is simple (e.g., linear), which may not correspond to the characteristics of the multi-modal data at hand [21]. To better account for the complexity of multi-modal data, other studies investigated *late fusion* strategies [19], where each modality is processed by an independent CNN and the multi-modal outputs are merged in a deep layer, as in the architecture depicted in Fig. 1, *middle*. This *late fusion* strategy was demonstrated to outperform *early fusion* on infant brain segmentation [19]. More recently, Aygün et al. explored different ways of combining multiple modalities [3]. In this work, all modalities are considered as separate inputs to different CNNs, which are later fused at an 'early', 'middle' or 'late' point. Although it was found that 'late' fusion provides better performance, as in [19], this method relies on a single-layer fusion to model the relation between all modalities. Nevertheless, as demonstrated in several works [21], relations between different modalities may be highly complex and cannot easily be modeled by a single layer. To account for the non-linearity in multi-modal data modeling, we recently proposed a CNN that incorporates dense connections not only between pairs of layers within the same path, but also between layers across different paths [9,11]. This architecture, known as *HyperDenseNet*, obtained very competitive performance in the context of infant and adult brain tissue segmentation with multi-modal MRI data.

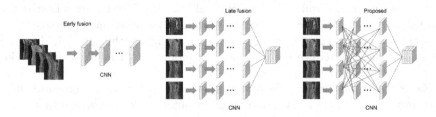

Fig. 1. Typical feature-fusion strategies (*left* and *middle*) and proposed fusion technique (*right*).

In the context of IVD localization and segmentation, Li et al. [17] have also considered multi-modal images. Specifically, they proposed a multi-scale and modality dropout learning framework, which employed four MRI modalities. To capture multi-scale context and handle the scale variations of IVDs, three different paths process regions extracted from the same location but at different scales. In addition, a random modality voxel dropout strategy is used to reduce feature co-adaptation between multiple modalities, and encourage each single modality to learn discriminative information independently.

Nevertheless, the combination of multi-modal data at various levels of abstraction has not been fully exploited for IVD localization and segmentation. In this work, we adopt the strategy presented in [9,11] and propose a multi-path architecture [8] called IVD-Net, where each modality is employed as input of one pathway, with dense connectivity used between the layers, within and across paths (Fig. 1, *right*). Furthermore, we extend the standard convolutional module of InceptionNet [22] by including two additional dilated convolutional blocks, which can help to learn larger context. In our previous work on multi-modal ischemic stroke lesion segmentation [8], we showed this model to outperform architectures based on early and late fusion, as well as several state-of-art segmentation networks.

2   Methodology

The proposed IVD-Net architecture follow the structure of UNet [20]. This well-known model is composed of two paths: one contracting and one expanding. While the former collapses the input image into a set of high level features forming a compact intermediate representation of the input, the latter employs these features to generate a pixel-wise segmentation mask. Furthermore, it includes skip-connections, which connect the outputs from shallow layers to the input of subsequent layers, with the goal of transferring information that may have been lost in the encoding path during the compression process.

2.1   Processing Multiple Modalities Separately

In order to fully exploit multi-modal data, we adopt the hyper-dense connectivity approach of [11] in the current work. To achieve this dense connectivity pattern, we first create an encoding path composed of multiple streams, each of them processing a different image modality. The main goal of employing separate streams for different modalities is to disentangle information that otherwise would be fused from an early stage, limiting the learning capabilities of the network to capture complex relationships between modalities. The structure of the proposed IVD-Net architecture is depicted in Fig. 2.

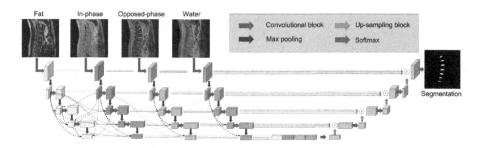

Fig. 2. Proposed IVD-Net architecture for IVD segmentation in multi-modal images, which extends the traditional UNet. Dotted lines represent some of the dense connectivity patterns adopted in this extended version of UNet.

2.2   Extended Inception Module

Meaningful areas in an image may undergo extremely large variation in size. In our particular case, as 3D segmentation is assessed in a 2D slice-wise manner, the region occupied by the IVD varies from one image to another. For instance, when the 2D sagittal slice corresponds to the center of the vertebral column, every IVD will appear in the image, whereas only one or two IVDs will be present in the image when the sagittal plane is located at extremes. This makes the selection of an accurate and general kernel size difficult. While a smaller kernel is better for local information, a larger kernel can capture information that is distributed globally. This idea is exploited in InceptionNet [22], where convolutions with multiple kernel sizes operate on the same level. Furthermore, in more recent versions, $n \times n$ convolutions are factorized to a combination of $1 \times n$ and $n \times 1$ convolutions, resulting in a 33% memory reduction.

To facilitate the learning of multiple contexts, we included two dilated convolutional blocks in parallel to the existing blocks in an inception module. Dilation rates of these blocks are different, which helps learning from different receptive fields, thereby increasing the context of the original inception modules. In addition, we removed max-pooling from the proposed architecture, as dilated convolutions were shown to be a better alternative, which captures more effectively the global context [25]. Our extended inception modules are depicted in Fig. 3.

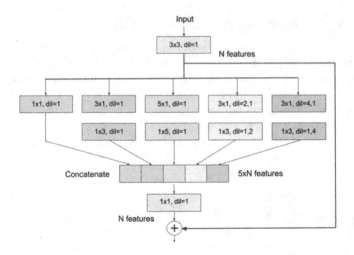

Fig. 3. Proposed extended inception modules. The module on the left employs standard convolutions while the module on the right adopts the idea of asymmetric convolutions [22].

2.3 Hyper-dense Connectivity

Inspired by the recent success of densely connected architectures for medical image segmentation [6,11,26], we adopted hyper-dense connections in the proposed model. The benefits of employing dense connections in the network are four-fold [11,13]. First, as demonstrated in [11], dense connections between multiple streams can better model relationships between different modalities. Second, flow of information and gradients through the entire network is facilitated by the use of direct connections between all layers, which alleviates the problem of vanishing gradient. Third, including short paths to all feature maps in the network introduces an implicit deep supervision. Fourth, dense connections have a regularizing effect, reducing the risk of over-fitting on tasks with smaller training sets.

Formulation. Let x_l denote the output of the lth layer, and H_l be a mapping function, which corresponds to a convolution layer followed by a non-linear activation. In standard CNNs, the output of the lth layer is typically obtained from the output of the previous layer x_{l-1} as

$$x_l = H_l(x_{l-1}). \tag{1}$$

In a densely-connected network, nevertheless, all feature outputs are concatenated in a feed-forward manner, i.e.,

$$x_l = H_l([x_{l-1}, x_{l-2}, \ldots, x_0]), \tag{2}$$

where [...] denotes a concatenation operation.

In the present work, as in HyperDenseNet [9,11], the outputs from previous layers in different streams are also concatenated to form the input of subsequent layers. This connectivity yields a much more powerful feature representation than early or late fusion strategies in a multi-modal context, as the network is capable of learning more complex relationships between the different modalities within and in-between all levels of abstraction. For simplicity, let us consider the scenario with only two modalities. Let x_l^1 and x_l^2 denote the outputs of the lth layer in streams 1 and 2, respectively. Then, the output of the lth layer in a given stream s can be defined as

$$x_l^s = H_l^s\left([x_{l-1}^1, x_{l-1}^2, x_{l-2}^1, x_{l-2}^2, \ldots, x_0^1, x_0^2]\right). \qquad (3)$$

Furthermore, recent works have found that shuffling and interleaving complete feature maps (or single feature maps elements) in a CNN can improve its performance, as it serves as a strong regularizer [7,28,30]. Inspired by this, we concatenate feature maps in a different order for each branch and layer, where the output of the lth layer now becomes

$$x_l^s = H_l^s\left(\pi_l^s([x_{l-1}^1, x_{l-1}^2, x_{l-2}^1, x_{l-2}^2, \ldots, x_0^1, x_0^2])\right), \qquad (4)$$

with π_l^s being a function that permutes the feature maps given as input. Thus, in the case of two image modalities, the outputs of the lth layers in both streams can be defined as

$$x_l^1 = H_l^1\left([x_{l-1}^1, x_{l-1}^2, x_{l-2}^1, x_{l-2}^2, \ldots, x_0^1, x_0^2]\right)$$
$$x_l^2 = H_l^2\left([x_{l-1}^2, x_{l-1}^1, x_{l-2}^2, x_{l-2}^1, \ldots, x_0^2, x_0^1]\right)$$

A detailed example of the adopted hyper-dense connectivity for the case of two image modalities is depicted in Fig. 4. This figure shows a section (only three levels) of a deep CNN where the two image modalities are processed in separated paths and modules are linked in a hyper-dense fashion.

3   Materials

3.1   Dataset

The provided IVD dataset is composed of 16 3D multi-modal MRI data sets of at least 7 IVDs of the lower spine, collected from 8 subjects in two different stages. Each MRI data set contains four aligned high-resolution 3D volumes: in-phase, opposed-phase, fat and water images. In addition to the MRI images, corresponding reference manual segmentations were provided. More detailed information about the dataset can be found at the IVD website[1].

---

[1] https://ivdm3seg.weebly.com.

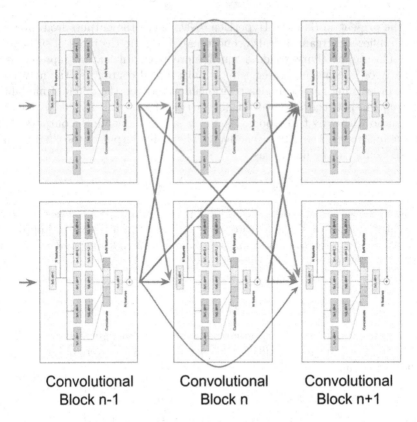

Fig. 4. Detailed version of a section of the proposed dense connectivity in multi-modal scenarios. For simplicity, two image modalities (in orange and in green) are considered in this example. While boxes represent a complete convolutional block of the proposed type, arrows indicate the connectivity pattern between modules. (Color figure online)

3.2 Evaluation Metrics

Even though segmentation is performed in a 2D-slice fashion, once all the 2D sagittal slices for a given patient have been segmented, they are stacked to reconstruct the original 3D volume. The metrics introduced below are therefore employed to evaluate performance on the whole 3D image. While the first metric is used to evaluate the segmentation accuracy, the second one serves as a measure of localization error.

Dice Similarity Coefficient (DSC). We first evaluate performance using Dice similarity coefficient (DSC), which compares volumes based on their overlap. Let V_{ref} and V_{auto} be the reference and automatic segmentations of a given tissue class and for a given subject, respectively. The DSC for this subject is defined as

$$\text{DSC}(V_{\text{ref}}, V_{\text{auto}}) = \frac{2 \mid V_{\text{ref}} \cap V_{\text{auto}} \mid}{\mid V_{\text{ref}} \mid + \mid V_{\text{auto}} \mid} \tag{5}$$

Localization Distance. To evaluate the localization error, we compute the 3D barycenters of ground-truth and predicted IVDs, and measure their Euclidean distance. Results are given in voxels.

3.3   Implementation Details

Baselines. Several architectures are used to demonstrate the effectiveness of the proposed network. As baselines, we consider two UNet versions, the first one with early fusion and the other with late fusion. In early fusion, following the procedure employed in most works, all MRI image modalities are merged into a single input which is processed through a unique path. In contrast, for late fusion, each MRI modality is processed in a separate stream, and learned features of different modalities are fused in a later stage. In both early and late fusion, the extended inception module of Fig. 3 is employed, however asymmetric convolutions are replaced by standard $n \times n$ convolutions in these baselines. Another difference with respect to standard UNet is that feature maps from skip connections are summed before being fed into convolutional modules of the decoding path, instead of being concatenated.

Proposed Network. In terms of architecture, the proposed IVD-Net network and the one employed with late fusion strategy are very similar. As introduced in Sect. 2.3, the main difference is that feature maps from previous layers and different paths are concatenated and fed into the subsequent layers, following Eq. (4). Details of the resulting architecture are provided in Table 1. The first version of the proposed network employs the same convolutional module as the two baselines, whereas the second version adopts asymmetric convolutions instead (Fig. 3).

Training. We employed Adam optimizer to train the proposed architectures, with $\beta_1 = 0.9$ and $\beta_2 = 0.99$. Training converged after 200 epochs with an initial learning rate of 1×10^{-4}, reduced by half after 100 epochs. Four images were used in each mini-batch. The same values for all hyper-parameters were employed across all architectures. Implementation of the analyzed architectures was done in PyTorch and experiments were performed on an NVidia TITAN XP GPU with 16 GBs RAM. While training was done in around 5 h, inference on a whole 3D volume took in 2–3 s on average. Images were normalized between 0 and 1 and no other pre- or post-processing steps were used. Furthermore, no data augmentation was employed to boost the performance of the networks. For all architectures, we used the four MRI modalities provided by the organizers as input. While 13 scans were employed for training 3 scans were used for validation.

4   Results

Quantitative results obtained with the different architectures are reported in Table 2. First, we observe that by simply fusing all image modalities at the input of the network provides the lowest mean DSC value. Adopting a late

Table 1. Layer placement of the proposed hyper-dense connected UNet.

	Name	HyperDense connectivity	
		Feat maps (input)	Feat maps (output)
Encoding Path (each modality)	Conv Layer 1	$1 \times 256 \times 256$	$32 \times 256 \times 256$
	Max-pooling 1	$32 \times 256 \times 256$	$32 \times 128 \times 128$
	Layer 2	$128 \times 128 \times 128$	$64 \times 128 \times 128$
	Max-pooling 2	$64 \times 128 \times 128$	$64 \times 64 \times 64$
	Layer 3	$384 \times 64 \times 64$	$128 \times 64 \times 64$
	Max-pooling 3	$128 \times 64 \times 64$	$128 \times 32 \times 32$
	Layer 4	$896 \times 32 \times 32$	$256 \times 32 \times 32$
	Max-pooling 4	$256 \times 32 \times 32$	$256 \times 16 \times 16$
	Bridge	$1920 \times 16 \times 16$	$512 \times 16 \times 16$
Decoding Path	Up-sample 1	$512 \times 16 \times 16$	$256 \times 32 \times 32$
	Layer 5	$256 \times 32 \times 32$	$256 \times 32 \times 32$
	Up-sample 2	$256 \times 32 \times 32$	$128 \times 64 \times 64$
	Layer 6	$128 \times 64 \times 64$	$128 \times 64 \times 64$
	Up-sample 3	$128 \times 64 \times 64$	$64 \times 128 \times 128$
	Layer 7	$64 \times 128 \times 128$	$64 \times 128 \times 128$
	Up-sample 4	$64 \times 128 \times 128$	$32 \times 256 \times 256$
	Layer 8	$32 \times 256 \times 256$	$32 \times 256 \times 256$
	Softmax layer	$32 \times 256 \times 256$	$2 \times 256 \times 256$

fusion strategy instead of early fusion achieves a mean DSC of 0.9086. Moreover, we see that our hyper-densely connected IVD-Net architecture brings a boost in performance compared to the more 'naive' early or late fusion strategies. When employing the extended module with standard convolutions (Fig. 3), we obtained a mean DSC of 0.9162, whereas the use of asymmetric convolutions in the proposed module provided the best performance in terms of mean DSC. These results are in line with values of localization distance, where the proposed architecture outperforms simpler fusion strategies. Nevertheless, in this case, the proposed network integrating standard convolutions slightly outperforms the architecture with asymmetric convolutions.

Table 2. Results on validation subjects obtained by the different architectures.

Architecture	DSC	Localization distance (voxels)
Baseline_EarlyFusion	0.8981 ± 0.0293	0.7701 ± 1.5872
Baseline_LateFusion	0.9086 ± 0.0339	0.7400 ± 1.6009
IVD-Net	0.9162 ± 0.0192	$\mathbf{0.4145 \pm 0.2698}$
IVD-Net (asym)	$\mathbf{0.9191 \pm 0.0179}$	0.4470 ± 0.2641

Qualitative evaluation of the proposed IVD-Net architecture is assessed in Figs. 5 and 6. First, ground truth and automatic contours obtained with IVD-Net are depicted on the sagittal plane in Fig. 5 for two validation subjects. Then, 3D rendered volumes for the ground truth and CNN segmentation are compared in Fig. 6. In both figures, we can see that the segmentation obtained by our architecture is very close to the manual annotated data, which aligns with the quantitative results in Table 2.

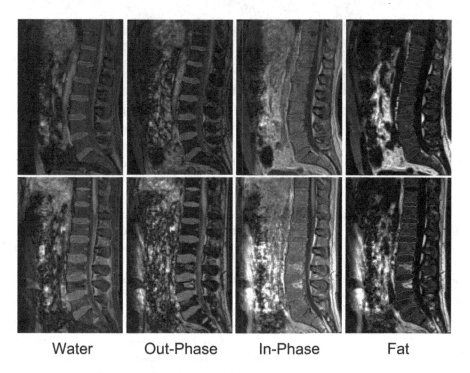

| Water | Out-Phase | In-Phase | Fat |

Fig. 5. Visual results for two subjects of the validation set. While the area in red represents the ground truth, bluish contours depict the automatic contours by our IVD-Net (asym) method in the different image modalities. (Color figure online)

5 Discussion

We have presented an architecture called IVD-Net that can efficiently leverage information from multiple image modalities for inter-vertebral disc segmentation. Following recent research on multi-modal image segmentation [8, 11], our architecture adopts dense connectivity between multiple paths in the encoding section, each of them processing single modalities. Specifically, convolutional layers in any stream receive as input the features maps of all previous layers in the same stream as well as from other streams.

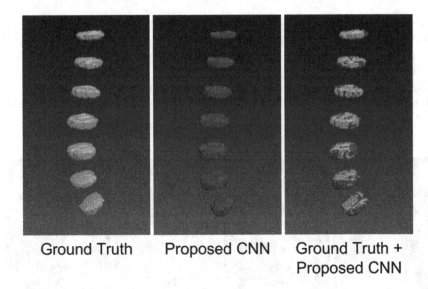

Ground Truth   Proposed CNN   Ground Truth +
                                     Proposed CNN

Fig. 6. 3D visualization of the ground truth, segmentation achieved by the proposed network and the combination of both for a subject on the validation set.

We have demonstrated that naive feature fusion strategies, such as simply merging information at an early or late stage, may be insufficient to fully exploit information in multi-modal scenarios. By allowing the network to learn how to combine learned features from separate modalities, it can capture more complex relationships between multiple sources. This improves its representation power, which ultimately results in a boost on performance. These findings are in line with recent works on multi-modal image segmentation [9,11,19]. For example, high-level features were combined at a late stage in [19], outperforming an early fusion strategy in the context of infant brain segmentation. In a recent work, we demonstrated that adopting more complex fusion techniques, referred to as hyper-dense connectivity, surpasses the performance of other features fusion strategies in the challenging tasks of infant and adult brain tissue segmentation [9,11].

Even though considering 3D context typically helps improve performance, we treated each volume as a stack of 2D sagittal slices (see Fig. 7). The main reason for this is that manual segmentations provided in this challenge were performed slice-wise in the sagittal plane. Thus, when looking at these annotations in the axial plane, a sharp contour is observed. As CNNs will generally provide a smooth contour, we assumed that tackling this problem as a 3D task would have led to lower values during evaluation. Furthermore, IVD localization is assessed after volumetric segmentation is done. This means that the process of localization itself is not optimized during training. A possible solution to overcome this limitation in the future might be to investigate multi-task architectures that can be trained end-to-end, so that both localization and segmentation tasks can be jointly optimized.

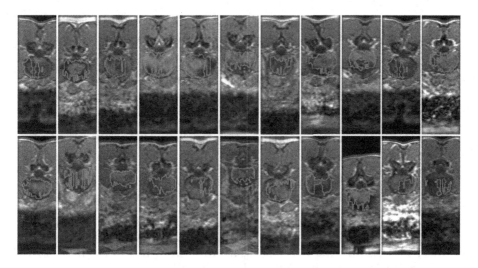

Fig. 7. Examples of manual annotations from the training set seen on axial slices.

Acknowledgments. This work is supported by the National Science and Engineering Research Council of Canada (NSERC), discovery grant program, and by the ETS Research Chair on Artificial Intelligence in Medical Imaging.

References

1. An, H.S., et al.: Introduction: disc degeneration: summary. Spine **29**(23), 2677–2678 (2004)
2. Ben Ayed, I., Punithakumar, K., Garvin, G., Romano, W., Li, S.: Graph cuts with invariant object-interaction priors: application to intervertebral disc segmentation. In: Székely, G., Hahn, H.K. (eds.) IPMI 2011. LNCS, vol. 6801, pp. 221–232. Springer, Heidelberg (2011). https://doi.org/10.1007/978-3-642-22092-0_19
3. Aygün, M., Şahin, Y.H., Ünal, G.: Multi modal convolutional neural networks forbrain tumor segmentation. arXiv preprint arXiv:1809.06191 (2018)
4. Chen, C., et al.: Localization and segmentation of 3D intervertebral discs in MR images by data driven estimation. IEEE Trans. Med. Imaging **34**(8), 1719–1729 (2015)
5. Chen, H., Dou, Q., Wang, X., Qin, J., Cheng, J.C.Y., Heng, P.-A.: 3D fully convolutional networks for intervertebral disc localization and segmentation. In: Zheng, G., Liao, H., Jannin, P., Cattin, P., Lee, S.-L. (eds.) MIAR 2016. LNCS, vol. 9805, pp. 375–382. Springer, Cham (2016). https://doi.org/10.1007/978-3-319-43775-0_34
6. Chen, L., Wu, Y., DSouza, A.M., Abidin, A.Z., Wismüller, A., Xu, C.: MRI tumor segmentation with densely connected 3D CNN. In: Medical Imaging 2018: Image Processing. International Society for Optics and Photonics (2018)
7. Chen, Y., Wang, H., Long, Y.: Regularization of convolutional neural networks using shufflenode. In: 2017 IEEE International Conference on Multimedia and Expo (ICME), pp. 355–360. IEEE (2017)

8. Dolz, J., Ben Ayed, I., Desrosiers, C.: Dense multi-path U-Net for ischemic stroke lesion segmentation in multiple image modalities. arXiv preprint arXiv:1810.07003 (2018)
9. Dolz, J., Ben Ayed, I., Yuan, J., Desrosiers, C.: Isointense infant brain segmentation with a hyper-dense connected convolutional neural network. In: 2018 IEEE 15th International Symposium on Biomedical Imaging, ISBI 2018, pp. 616–620. IEEE (2018)
10. Dolz, J., Desrosiers, C., Wang, L., Yuan, J., Shen, D., Ben Ayed, I.: Deep CNN ensembles and suggestive annotations for infant brain MRI segmentation. arXiv preprint arXiv:1712.05319, 2017
11. Dolz, J., Gopinath, K., Yuan, J., Lombaert, H., Desrosiers, C., Ben Ayed, I.: HyperDense-Net: a hyper-densely connected CNN for multi-modal image segmentation. In: IEEE Transactions on Medical Imaging (2018, in press)
12. Hamanishi, C., Matukura, N., Fujita, M., Tomihara, M., Tanaka, S.: Cross-sectional area of the stenotic lumbar dural tube measured from the transverse views of magnetic resonance imaging. J. Spinal Disord. **7**(5), 388–393 (1994)
13. Huang, G., Liu, Z., Van Der Maaten, L., Weinberger, K.Q.: Densely connected convolutional networks. In: CVPR, vol. 1, p. 3 (2017)
14. Ji, X., Zheng, G., Belavy, D., Ni, D.: Automated intervertebral disc segmentation using deep convolutional neural networks. In: Yao, J., Vrtovec, T., Zheng, G., Frangi, A., Glocker, B., Li, S. (eds.) CSI 2016. LNCS, vol. 10182, pp. 38–48. Springer, Cham (2016). https://doi.org/10.1007/978-3-319-55050-3_4
15. Kamnitsas, K., et al.: Efficient multi-scale 3D CNN with fully connected CRF for accurate brain lesion segmentation. Med. Image Anal. **36**, 61–78 (2017)
16. Kim, S., Bae, W., Masuda, K., Chung, C., Hwang, D.: Fine-grain segmentation of the intervertebral discs from MR spine images using deep convolutional neural networks: BSU-Net. Appl. Sci. **8**(9), 1656 (2018)
17. Li, X., et al.: 3D multi-scale FCN with random modality voxel dropout learning for intervertebral disc localization and segmentation from multi-modality MR images. Med. Image Anal. **45**, 41–54 (2018)
18. Moeskops, P., Viergever, M.A., Mendrik, A.M., de Vries, L.S., Benders, M.J., Išgum, I.: Automatic segmentation of MR brain images with a convolutional neural network. IEEE Trans. Med. Imaging **35**(5), 1252–1261 (2016)
19. Nie, D., Wang, L., Gao, Y., Sken, D.: Fully convolutional networks for multi-modality isointense infant brain image segmentation. In: 13th International Symposium on Biomedical Imaging (ISBI), pp. 1342–1345. IEEE (2016)
20. Ronneberger, O., Fischer, P., Brox, T.: U-Net: convolutional networks for biomedical image segmentation. In: Navab, N., Hornegger, J., Wells, W.M., Frangi, A.F. (eds.) MICCAI 2015. LNCS, vol. 9351, pp. 234–241. Springer, Cham (2015). https://doi.org/10.1007/978-3-319-24574-4_28
21. Srivastava, N., Salakhutdinov, R.: Multimodal learning with deep boltzmann machines. J. Mach. Learn. Res. **15**, 2949–2980 (2014)
22. Szegedy, C., Vanhoucke, V., Ioffe, S., Shlens, J., Wojna, Z.: Rethinking the inception architecture for computer vision. In: CVPR, pp. 2818–2826 (2016)
23. Valverde, S., et al.: Improving automated multiple sclerosis lesion segmentation with a cascaded 3D convolutional neural network approach. NeuroImage **155**, 159–168 (2017)
24. Wieser, S., et al.: Cost of low back pain in switzerland in 2005. Eur. J. Health Econ. **12**(5), 455–467 (2011)
25. Yu, F., Koltun, V.: Multi-scale context aggregation by dilated convolutions. arXiv preprint arXiv:1511.07122 (2015)

26. Yu, L., et al.: Automatic 3D cardiovascular MR segmentation with densely-connected volumetric ConvNets. In: Descoteaux, M., Maier-Hein, L., Franz, A., Jannin, P., Collins, D.L., Duchesne, S. (eds.) MICCAI 2017. LNCS, vol. 10434, pp. 287–295. Springer, Cham (2017). https://doi.org/10.1007/978-3-319-66185-8_33
27. Zeng, G., Zheng, G.: DSMS-FCN: a deeply supervised multi-scale fully convolutional network for automatic segmentation of intervertebral disc in 3D MR images. In: Glocker, B., Yao, J., Vrtovec, T., Frangi, A., Zheng, G. (eds.) MSKI 2017. LNCS, vol. 10734, pp. 148–159. Springer, Cham (2018). https://doi.org/10.1007/978-3-319-74113-0_13
28. Zhang, T., Qi, G.-J., Xiao, B., Wang, J.: Interleaved group convolutions. In: CVPR, pp. 4373–4382 (2017)
29. Zhang, W., et al.: Deep convolutional neural networks for multi-modality isointense infant brain image segmentation. NeuroImage **108**, 214–224 (2015)
30. Zhang, X., Zhou, X., Lin, M., Sun, J.: Shufflenet: an extremely efficient convolutional neural network for mobile devices. arXiv preprint arXiv:1707.01083 (2017)
31. Zheng, G., et al.: Evaluation and comparison of 3D intervertebral disc localization and segmentation methods for 3D T2 MR data: a grand challenge. Med. Image Anal. **35**, 327–344 (2017)

Intervertebral Disc Segmentation and Localization from Multi-modality MR Images with 2.5D Multi-scale Fully Convolutional Network and Geometric Constraint Post-processing

Chang Liu[1,2] and Liang Zhao[1(✉)]

[1] SenseTime, Beijing, China
liu.luckpp@gmail.com, zhaoliang@sensetime.com
[2] Institute for Medical Imaging Technology, School of Biomedical Engineering,
Shanghai Jiao Tong University, Shanghai, China

Abstract. The intervertebral discs (IVDs) segmentation and localization on medical images are important for the clinical diagnosis and research of spine diseases. In this work, we proposed a robust automatic method based on 2.5D multi-scale fully convolutional network (FCN) and geometric constraint post-processing for IVD segmentation and localization on 3D multi-modality Magnetic Resonance (MR) scans. Firstly, we designed a 2.5D multi-scale FCN. And the ensemble outputs of such three networks are used as the IVD prediction maps. The final segmentation and localization of IVDs are generated from these prediction maps with a geometric constraint post-processing method. This work ranked the first in the on-site test of MICCAI 2018 Challenge on Automatic Intervertebral Disc Localization and Segmentation from 3D Multi-modality MR Images (IVDM3Seg).

Keywords: Intervertebral disc · Segmentation · Localization ·
Fully convolutional network

1 Introduction

The intervertebral disc (IVD) is a cartilaginous joint that lies between adjacent vertebras. It plays a crucial role in the shock absorption of vertebral movement [1, 2]. In modern society, back pain is becoming a common healthy problem, which causes the pain, stiffness and loss of independency of patients. According to the international studies, the point prevalence of back pain is between 12% and 35%, while the lifetime prevalence is up to 49% to 80% [3]. For this disease, degeneration of the intervertebral disc is considered as a major cause [4].

Magnetic Resonance Imaging (MRI) is a commonly used imaging technique in the diagnosis of IVD degeneration and many other diseases, which provides non-invasive assessment to human body. Compared to other medical imaging methods, such as Computed Tomography (CT) imaging, MRI could provide excellent contrast in soft

© Springer Nature Switzerland AG 2019
G. Zheng et al. (Eds.): CSI 2018, LNCS 11397, pp. 144–153, 2019.
https://doi.org/10.1007/978-3-030-13736-6_12

tissue without ionizing radiation. Besides, the MR scans could be obtained with different modalities, and provide more information about tissue structure. In this work, four MRI modalities (i.e. in-phase, opposed-phase, water, fat) were used for the segmentation and localization of IVDs. Figure 1 shows an example of these four modalities. It should be noticed that only the 7 IVDs between the twelfth thoracic vertebra and sacrum are delineated manually as the targets.

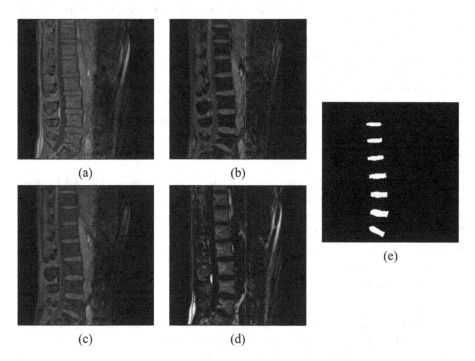

Fig. 1. An example of 3D multi-modality images provided by MICCAI 2018 Challenge on IVDM3Seg. (a) to (d) are in-phase, opposed-phase, water, and fat modality in order while (e) is the manually delineated labels for 7 IVDs between the twelfth thoracic vertebra and sacrum.

The research on IVD degeneration usually needs the segmentation of IVDs. Traditionally, the IVD labels are delineated manually. However, this job is always time-consuming and may be biased for inter- and intra-observer variabilities [5, 6]. For this matter, automatic IVD segmentation and localization methods have great significance to the study of IVD degeneration.

There are three main challenges for automatic IVD segmentation and localization on multi-modality images. Firstly, distinguishing different IVDs is difficult due to the intra-subject similarity of IVDs. Secondly, the intensity of IVD boundary resembles that of the neighborhood tissues, which makes the IVD contour fuzzy. Thirdly, how to harness the multi-modality information effectively in medical image processing remains to be explored.

1.1 Previous Work

There are many segmentation and localization methods proposed in previous research, which are based on traditional hand-crafted features [7–13]. Besides, some popular graph-based methods, such as graph cut [10] and statistical shape model [7], were also applied to IVD segmentation. For localization, some graphical models were proposed to take IVD geometric relationship into account [13]. With the reference to the local parts shape and neighborhood anatomical structures, the accuracy of IVD localization improved in some degree.

In recent years, machine learning has drawn extensive attention in many fields. Some classical machine learning algorithms, such as marginal space learning (MSL) [14], Adaboost [15], and sparse kernel machine [16], were also adopted to IVD segmentation and localization. And these methods have shown excellent performance.

More recently, deep learning techniques achieved great success in computer vision. Many researchers began to attempt deep learning algorithms in medical image processing. And these methods have proven effective. In the past few years, all the state-of-art methods on MICCAI IVD segmentation and localization challenge were deep learning-based [17, 18].

Multi-modality images are not only available for IVD segmentation and localization. How to utilize multi-modality information is a common issue in medical image processing, such as MRI-based brain tissue [19] and brain tumor segmentation [20]. Generally, the harness of multi-modality data could improve the performance more or less.

1.2 Our Contribution

We propose a 2.5D multi-scale deep learning network for segmentation and localization of IVDs on multi-modality MR scans. Our method achieved the state-of-art performance in the MICCAI 2018 Challenge on IVDM3Seg.

Our main contributions are summarized below:

1. We proposed a multi-scale 2.5D fully convolutional network (FCN) for IVD segmentation and localization on multi-modality MR scans. The back bone of the proposed network is a U-Net [21] like architecture. The input of the 2.5D network is a few adjacent slices from multi-modality MR scans, while the output of this network is a 2D slice corresponding to a certain layer of the input. For the purpose of make full advantage of multi-modality information, Squeeze-and-Excitation (SE) modules [22] are added in the skip connections.
2. We proposed a model fusion strategy to improve accuracy and robustness of IVD prediction. In this work, we trained three different 2.5D networks. The predictions of these models are corresponding to the middle, the rightmost, and the leftmost slices of the input sequence. For the slices located at the middle of 3D images along Z-axis, the average outputs of these models are taken as the final predictions. For the slices near the both edges, IVD predictions are generated by the model, which is corresponding to either the rightmost or the leftmost slice of the input sequence.
3. We proposed a geometric constraint post-processing method to generate accurate IVD localization results. This method takes the intra-subject geometric relationship

of IVDs into account. In our experiments, the false positive regions on the prediction maps are well eliminated by this method.

2 Methodology

The detail of IVD segmentation and localization method is elaborated in this section. We start by illustrating the architecture of proposed 2.5D multi-scale FCN for IVD segmentation. Furthermore, we explain the way to harness multi-modality images with this network. To improve the robustness and accuracy of prediction, an ensemble strategy is employed in this work. In order to correct the false positive regions in prediction maps, we proposed a post-processing pipeline, which takes geometric constraint of 7 specified IVDs into account. The final results of segmentation and localization are generated by this post-processing method.

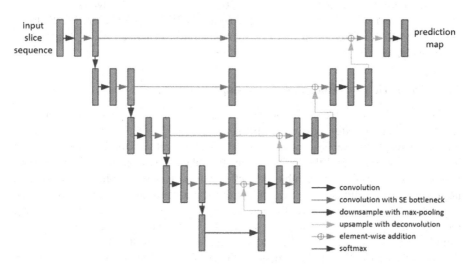

Fig. 2. The details of our proposed 2.5D multi-scale FCN for IVD segmentation. The input slice sequence includes 44 slices, which consists of 11 consecutive slices from four modalities with the same corresponding position. The prediction map is corresponding to the middle, the leftmost, or the right most slice of the input sequence.

2.1 2.5D Multi-scale FCN for IVD Segmentation

The detail structure of proposed network is shown in Fig. 2. The back bone of this network is a U-Net like architecture, which has achieved great success in medical image processing since it was proposed in 2015. To utilize multi-modality images, the architecture of U-Net is slightly adapted from the origin version. The input of this network is expanded up to 44 (11 slices * 4 modalities) channels to harness the multi-modality data, while the output is corresponding to a certain position of the input sequence. Besides, residual connections are added between feature maps with the same scale. And SE modules are also inserted in skip connections between the contracting path and the expansive path. The reduction ratio used in SE modules is set to be 16.

2.2   2.5D Multi-scale FCN Ensemble Strategy

All the multi-modality images used in this work are in the same size of 256 * 256 * 36. For each study, 11 consecutive slices from four modalities with the same corresponding position are extracted and concatenated as the input sequences. And there are 26 such consecutive sequences for each image. These input sequences are utilized to train three 2.5D multi-scale FCNs. The prediction of these models is corresponding to different layers respectively, which are the middle, the leftmost and the rightmost slices in the input sequence. We use m_{middle}, m_{left} and m_{right} to denote these three models in the following content. The ensemble outputs of these models are produced as prediction results, which are more accurate and robust. For the simplicity of description, a mono-modality 3D image V is picked as an example. Slices in V from left to right are denoted as $S_i (i \in \{1, 2, \ldots, 26\})$. For S_6 to S_{31}, the average outputs of m_{middle}, m_{left} and m_{right} are taken as the prediction of IVD segmentation. For S_1 to S_5 and S_{32} to S_{36}, the prediction of IVD segmentation is generated by m_{left} and m_{right} respectively.

2.3   Geometric Constraint Post-processing

Although model ensemble can improve the accuracy and robustness of segmentation results to a certain extent, there are still some obvious false positive regions in the prediction maps. These false positive areas could be categorized as two types, the isolated noise points, and the IVD segmentation above the twelfth thoracic vertebra. Figure 3 visualizes some ensemble prediction maps on opposed-phase. The isolated noise can be well eliminated by excluding the small connected regions in prediction maps. For IVDs above the twelfth thoracic vertebra, we proposed a post-processing method with geometric constraint for removal. Firstly, we picked the ground truths from training set, and aligned them to the segmentation result with reference to the centroid of the last IVD. These ground truths are then registered to the segmentation result with affine transformation. The best fitted one is then selected as the mask. Remove all the connected regions that have no intersection with this mask. The remaining content is right the final prediction of 7 expected IVDs. For the robustness of post-processing, the registered ground truth was dilated before being applied as the mask (Fig. 4).

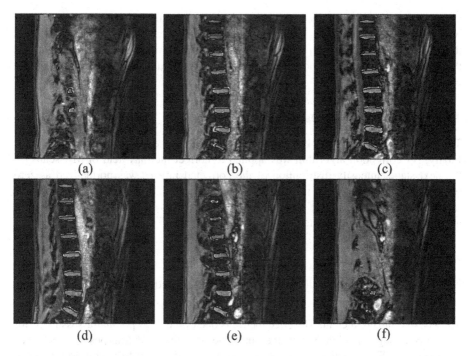

Fig. 3. Examples of prediction map on opposed-phase without post-processing. (a) to (f) are 6 slices extracted from a study. Green contours indicate the boundary of the ground truths. And the ensemble prediction of IVDs is delineated by red lines. (Color figure online)

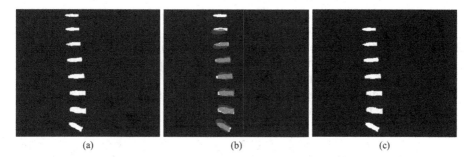

Fig. 4. Illustration of the geometric constraint post-processing. (a) is the ensemble prediction of proposed networks. The red mask in (b) is the chosen registered ground truth with binary dilation. And (c) is the final IVD segmentation result of our method. (Color figure online)

3 Experiments and Results

3.1 Data

The performance of our method was evaluated on multi-modality MR scans provided by MICCAI 2018 Challenge on IVDM3Seg. These data were collected from 8 subjects at two time points of prolonged bed rest study. For each study, four MR scans acquired with different modalities (i.e. in-phase, opposed-phase, water, fat) were enrolled. And the IVDs between the twelfth thoracic vertebra and sacrum are delineated manually as the ground truth. Figure 1 shows an example of these multi-modality images and the corresponding ground truth.

3.2   Pre-processing and Data Augmentation

The multi-modality images were pre-processed with some commonly used methods. Firstly, N4 correction algorithm was applied to correct the bias field of MR scans. In the next stage, intensity distribution of the corrected images was normalized as zero mean and unit variance. For the inadequacy of training data, some data augmentation methods (i.e. random scale, rotate, translation, and deformable transformation) are applied during the training stage.

3.3   Evaluation Metrics

The segmentation and localization results are evaluated with the following three quantitative metrics:

1. Dice overlap coefficient. The Dice metric is one of the most popular assessments for semantic segmentation, which measures the percentage of true positive voxels in prediction. The definition of Dice can be expressed by the following formula:

$$Dice = \frac{2|A \cap B|}{|A| \cap |B|} \times 100\% \tag{1}$$

Where A is the set of foreground voxels in the ground truth and B denotes the corresponding set in the prediction of foreground.

2. Average absolute distance (ASD). For IVD segmentation task, ASD is the average absolute distance between disc surface of ground truth and segmentation result. Smaller ASD means a better segmentation result.

3. Localization distance. This metric is used for measuring the localization results. It is calculated by the equation below:

$$R = \sqrt{(\Delta x)^2 + (\Delta y)^2 + (\Delta z)^2} \tag{2}$$

Where Δx, Δy and Δz are the absolute distance between the identified IVD centroids and the corresponding ground truth along X-, Y- and Z-axis. It is obvious that a smaller localization distance means a more accurate localization.

3.4   Results of MICCAI 2018 On-site Challenge

Tables 1, 2, and 3 list the on-site test results of MICCAI 2018 Challenge on IVDM3Seg with proposed method. Our method achieved the state-of-art performance with the respect of all the three quantitative metrics (i.e. Dice, ASD, and Localization distance) among nine participating teams.

Table 1. Dice of on-site test results

Dice	Disc_01	Disc_02	Disc_03	Disc_04	Disc_05	Disc_06	Disc_07
Test_01	0.887	0.904	0.927	0.911	0.896	0.890	0.869
Test_02	0.909	0.934	0.941	0.944	0.930	0.925	0.924
Test_03	0.896	0.898	0.901	0.866	0.896	0.817	0.887
Test_04	0.920	0.939	0.938	0.915	0.912	0.885	0.924
Test_05	0.900	0.911	0.917	0.918	0.868	0.898	0.926
Test_06	0.865	0.914	0.930	0.909	0.897	0.898	0.892
Test_07	0.905	0.931	0.931	0.915	0.904	0.890	0.865
Test_08	0.905	0.928	0.924	0.925	0.910	0.907	0.889

Table 2. ASD of on-site test results

ASD (mm)	Disc_01	Disc_02	Disc_03	Disc_04	Disc_05	Disc_06	Disc_07
Test_01	0.73	0.67	0.49	0.58	0.63	0.61	0.67
Test_02	0.54	0.48	0.43	0.37	0.43	0.41	0.41
Test_03	0.71	0.80	0.73	0.87	0.58	0.89	0.53
Test_04	0.54	0.47	0.41	0.49	0.47	0.51	0.29
Test_05	0.57	0.70	0.69	0.61	0.98	0.67	0.37
Test_06	0.85	0.66	0.56	0.76	0.78	0.69	0.54
Test_07	0.63	0.52	0.52	0.63	0.62	0.64	0.64
Test_08	0.72	0.63	0.61	0.57	0.62	0.57	0.58

Table 3. Localization distance of on-site test results

Localization (mm)	Disc_01	Disc_02	Disc_03	Disc_04	Disc_05	Disc_06	Disc_07
Test_01	0.41	1.42	0.52	0.78	1.37	1.02	1.09
Test_02	0.30	0.73	0.27	0.50	0.72	0.40	0.17
Test_03	0.64	0.31	1.34	2.12	0.97	1.30	0.43
Test_04	0.81	0.52	0.62	1.30	0.49	1.22	0.08
Test_05	0.79	0.30	0.13	1.02	0.92	0.97	0.41
Test_06	1.23	0.47	0.45	0.09	0.65	1.09	0.76
Test_07	0.56	1.09	0.94	1.22	1.19	0.58	1.08
Test_08	0.36	1.31	0.72	0.91	1.04	0.34	0.56

4 Discussion

Some common spine diseases, such as low back pain (LBP), have proven to be associated with IVD degeneration [23]. IVD segmentation and localization have important significance in clinical diagnosis and research. In this work, we proposed an automatic IVD segmentation and localization method on multi-modality MRI with 2.5D multi-scale FCN and geometric constraint post-processing.

In the MICCAI 2018 Challenge on IVDM3Seg, the deep neural network is the most popular algorithm. For 3D multi-modality MR images, processing with a 3D network is a straightforward approach. Compared to 2D networks, 3D architectures could generate more discriminative spatial features. And these architectures were employed by some teams in this challenge. Due to the plenty of parameters in deep neural networks, a huge amount of data is demanded in training stage. However, there were only 16 studies provided by MICCAI 2018 Challenge on IVDM3Seg, which were collected from 8 subjects at two time points. Considering the inadequacy of 3D multi-modality images, we proposed a 2.5D multi-scale FCN architecture as a tradeoff between the capacity of network and the amount of training data. The on-site test results of MICCAI 2018 Challenge on IVDM3Seg shows that the performance of 2D networks was better than that of 3D networks in general with limited training data. And our 2.5D FCN surpassed both 2D and 3D architectures.

The intra-subject morphology and topology relationship between IVDs are similar inter-subjects. And it is potential to be utilized for IVD localization. However, this relationship is hard to be captured by FCN. To take this information into account, we proposed a geometric constraint post-processing method based on registration. And it shows great performance in on-site test of MICCAI 2018 Challenge on IVDM3Seg. It should be noticed that our registration-based post-processing relies on the inter-subject consistency of IVD intra-subject geometric relationship. If this consistency was destroyed by some severe spine diseases, this method may produce wrong cases. The IVD localization method with better robustness remains to be explored in the future work.

References

1. An, H.S., et al.: Introduction: disc degeneration: summary. Spine 29, 2677–2678 (2004)
2. Urban, J.P., Roberts, S.J.A.R.T.: Degeneration of the intervertebral disc. Arthritis Res. Ther. 5, 120 (2003)
3. Maniadakis, N., Gray, A.J.P.: The economic burden of back pain in the UK. Pain 84, 95–103 (2000)
4. Luoma, K., Riihimäki, H., Luukkonen, R., Raininko, R., Viikari-Juntura, E., Lamminen, A.J.S.: Low back pain in relation to lumbar disc degeneration. Spine 25, 487–492 (2000)
5. Niemeläinen, R., Videman, T., Dhillon, S., Battié, M.: Quantitative measurement of intervertebral disc signal using MRI. Clin. Radiol. 63, 252–255 (2008)
6. Violas, P., Estivalezes, E., Briot, J., de Gauzy, J.S., Swider, P.: Objective quantification of intervertebral disc volume properties using MRI in idiopathic scoliosis surgery. Magn. Reson. Imaging 25, 386–391 (2007)
7. Neubert, A., et al.: Automated 3D segmentation of vertebral bodies and intervertebral discs from MRI. In: 2011 International Conference on Digital Image Computing Techniques and Applications (DICTA), pp. 19–24 (2011)

8. Corso, J.J., Alomari, R.S., Chaudhary, V.: Lumbar disc localization and labeling with a probabilistic model on both pixel and object features. In: Metaxas, D., Axel, L., Fichtinger, G., Székely, G. (eds.) MICCAI 2008. LNCS, vol. 5241, pp. 202–210. Springer, Heidelberg (2008). https://doi.org/10.1007/978-3-540-85988-8_25

9. Chevrefils, C., Chériet, F., Grimard, G., Aubin, C.-E.: Watershed segmentation of intervertebral disk and spinal canal from MRI images. In: Kamel, M., Campilho, A. (eds.) ICIAR 2007. LNCS, vol. 4633, pp. 1017–1027. Springer, Heidelberg (2007). https://doi.org/10.1007/978-3-540-74260-9_90

10. Ben Ayed, I., Punithakumar, K., Garvin, G., Romano, W., Li, S.: Graph cuts with invariant object-interaction priors: application to intervertebral disc segmentation. In: Székely, G., Hahn, H.K. (eds.) IPMI 2011. LNCS, vol. 6801, pp. 221–232. Springer, Heidelberg (2011). https://doi.org/10.1007/978-3-642-22092-0_19

11. Raja'S, A., Corso, J.J., Chaudhary, V.: Labeling of lumbar discs using both pixel-and object-level features with a two-level probabilistic model. IEEE Trans. Med. Imaging **30**, 1–10 (2011)

12. Chevrefils, C., Cheriet, F., Aubin, C.É., Grimard, G.: Texture analysis for automatic segmentation of intervertebral disks of scoliotic spines from MR images. IEEE Trans. Inf Technol. Biomed. **13**, 608–620 (2009)

13. Schmidt, S., et al.: Spine detection and labeling using a parts-based graphical model. In: Karssemeijer, N., Lelieveldt, B. (eds.) IPMI 2007. LNCS, vol. 4584, pp. 122–133. Springer, Heidelberg (2007). https://doi.org/10.1007/978-3-540-73273-0_11

14. Kelm, B.M., et al.: Spine detection in CT and MR using iterated marginal space learning. Med. Image Anal. **17**, 1283–1292 (2013)

15. Huang, S.-H., Chu, Y.-H., Lai, S.-H., Novak, C.L.: Learning-based vertebra detection and iterative normalized-cut segmentation for spinal MRI. IEEE Trans. Med. Imaging **28**, 1595–1605 (2009)

16. Wang, Z., Zhen, X., Tay, K., Osman, S., Romano, W., Li, S.: Regression segmentation for M^3 spinal images. IEEE Trans. Med. Imaging **34**, 1640–1648 (2015)

17. Li, X., et al.: 3D multi-scale FCN with random modality voxel dropout learning for Intervertebral Disc Localization and Segmentation from Multi-modality MR Images. Med. Image Anal. **45**, 41–54 (2018)

18. Chen, H., Dou, Q., Wang, X., Qin, J., Cheng, J.C.Y., Heng, P.-A.: 3D fully convolutional networks for intervertebral disc localization and segmentation. In: Zheng, G., Liao, H., Jannin, P., Cattin, P., Lee, S.-L. (eds.) MIAR 2016. LNCS, vol. 9805, pp. 375–382. Springer, Cham (2016). https://doi.org/10.1007/978-3-319-43775-0_34

19. Zhang, W., et al.: Deep convolutional neural networks for multi-modality isointense infant brain image segmentation. NeuroImage **108**, 214–224 (2015)

20. Havaei, M., Guizard, N., Chapados, N., Bengio, Y.: HeMIS: hetero-modal image segmentation. In: Ourselin, S., Joskowicz, L., Sabuncu, M.R., Unal, G., Wells, W. (eds.) MICCAI 2016. LNCS, vol. 9901, pp. 469–477. Springer, Cham (2016). https://doi.org/10.1007/978-3-319-46723-8_54

21. Ronneberger, O., Fischer, P., Brox, T.: U-Net: convolutional networks for biomedical image segmentation. In: Navab, N., Hornegger, J., Wells, W.M., Frangi, A.F. (eds.) MICCAI 2015. LNCS, vol. 9351, pp. 234–241. Springer, Cham (2015). https://doi.org/10.1007/978-3-319-24574-4_28

22. Hu, J., Shen, L., Sun, G.: Squeeze-and-excitation networks. arXiv preprint arXiv:1709. 01507, vol. 7 (2017)

23. Kjaer, P., Leboeuf-Yde, C., Korsholm, L., Sorensen, J.S., Bendix, T.: Magnetic resonance imaging and low back pain in adults: a diagnostic imaging study of 40-year-old men and women. Spine **30**, 1173–1180 (2005)

Automatic Segmentation of Lumbar Spine MRI Using Ensemble of 2D Algorithms

Nedelcho Georgiev[✉] and Asen Asenov[✉]

SmartSoft Ltd., Gen.Kolev 113, suite 7.3, 9000 Varna, Bulgaria
{nedelcho.georgiev,asen.asenov}@smart-soft.net

Abstract. MRI is considered the gold standard in soft tissue diagnostic of the lumbar spine. Number of protocols and modalities are used – from one hand 2D sagittal, 2D angulated axial, 2D consecutive axial and 3D image types; from the other hand different sequences and contrasts are used: T1w, T2w; fat suppression, water suppression etc. Images of different modalities are not always aligned. Resolutions and field of view also vary. SNR is also different for different MRI equipment. So the goal should be to create an algorithm that covers great variety of imaging techniques.

1 Introduction

MRI is considered the gold standard in soft tissue diagnostic of the lumbar spine. Number of protocols and modalities are used – from one hand 2D sagittal, 2D angulated axial, 2D consecutive axial and 3D image types; from the other hand different sequences and contrasts are used: T1w, T2w; fat suppression, water suppression etc. Images of different modalities are not always aligned. Resolutions and field of view also vary. SNR is also different for different MRI equipment. So the goal should be to create an algorithm that covers great variety of imaging techniques.

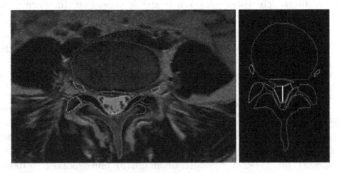

Fig. 1. (a) Segmentation of axial T2w slide; (b) Measurement of dural sac in a different slide (white line).

We consider the segmentation as the first step in a 3-step process: 1. Segmentation Fig. 1(a); 2. Measurements Fig. 1(b); 3. Diagnosis (in the case shown in the Fig. 1(b) -

© Springer Nature Switzerland AG 2019
G. Zheng et al. (Eds.): CSI 2018, LNCS 11397, pp. 154–162, 2019.
https://doi.org/10.1007/978-3-030-13736-6_13

severity of disk herniation and central canal stenosis grading). Our system detects most of the visible tissues that are relevant for diagnosing a pathology. One of the tissues is Intervertebral Discs. We applied our method with some extensions to detect intervertebral discs in the IVDM3Seg Segmentation Challenge [7].

2 Methods

In order to cover different protocols a 2D single modality algorithm was developed that in cases of 3D multi-modality data can be used in ensemble of multiple 2D single modality data models. Our 2D algorithms are using CNN [1] and are greatly inspired of ResNet [2]. Dropout regularization [3] and batch normalizations [4] are also used. FCN [5] style network is used for the super-pixel classification as this enable arbitrary field of view input. Super-pixels are 8 times smaller (in all dimensions) than the actual pixels (as stride 8 is used due to 3 2×2 max pooling layers). As a result fine grained details are lost, so we use Unet-like [6] architecture for up-scaling the low resolution map into the resolution of the input image. Separate 2D single modality results are combined into 3D results using ensemble with learnable weights combining the 3D information from 3 separate probability maps. To overcome the problem with small data set size, extensive augmentations were used: crop and resize, tilt, rotate, dynamic range changes, random noise in all possible combinations.

Datasets. Our dataset consists of 30 patient studies, 918 axial and sagittal slices in total. The patients' age ranges from 30 to 50 years old, with a mean age of 37.5 years old, including both male and female patients suffering from lower back pain. This data was provided by three medical centers, two of which use a GE Medical Systems to acquire MRI. The third set of MRI was acquired by a SIEMENS machine. The characteristics of the slices in the dataset vary:

- Voxel Thickness: 3.5 mm to 10 mm (mean 7.4 mm)
- Repetition Time: from 1040 ms to 6739 ms
- Echo Time: from 9.6 ms to 110.3 ms
- Axial Resolutions (Cols $\times$ Rows): 512×512, 276×192
- Sagittal Resolutions (Cols $\times$ Rows): 512×512, 384×768.

The slices are not uniformly spaced and are not parallel to each other. The axial slices are parallel to each of the discs. This way there is no value for each of the voxels in the volume of the study. 3D ensemble from this data set is not straight forward The challenge dataset provided by IVDM3seg consisting of 16 patients with full 3D data available, consisting of 4 modalities.

Feature Extraction. Fully convolutional ResNet-50 was used for feature map extractor. The model is pretrained on COCO. The minimal stride of the feature map for pretrained model we could find was 8. For Image ($512 \times 512 \times 3$) a feature map ($64 \times 64 \times 1024$) is produced. It is believed that the bigger feature stride causes lower resolution imperfections in the masks. For 256 * 256 * 37 the smallest feature map resolution is 4. An attempt to overcome this limitation was UNet-like mask predictor architecture.

The model originally uses 3 input channels (RGB). To make use of the modalities of the MRI, the 3 most useful modalities are used as input in the feature extractor model (Fig. 2).

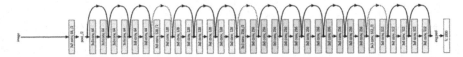

Fig. 2. The ResNet

Segmentation. To produce more accurate masks, which capture finer detail and higher frequency changes in the contour, a UNet-like architecture was used. To produce the mask, series of up-convolutions are used, starting from the stride 8 feature maps of the feature extractor and doubling the resolution on each layer. Each layer is combined with the corresponding resolution feature map from an internal layer in the feature extractor. This way higher level, lower resolution semantic features are used as context, and lower level, higher resolution features are used for finer details (Fig. 3).

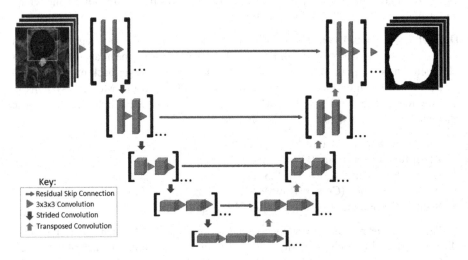

Fig. 3. The UNet-like segmentation architecture

3D Ensemble. The prediction from 3 2D models (axial, sagittal, coronal) are combined using a 3D convolution neural network. It has 2 layers of $3 \times 3 \times 3$ convolutions that are trained on the predictions of one part of the validation set and validated on the other part. The challenge data set is divided into train and validation set. The 3 models are trained on the train set and the hyper parameters are tuned on the validation set. When the models are trained one part of the validation set is predicted and the predicted probability maps are used to train the 3D convolution model.

The input for the 3D convolution is 6 channel 3D matrix. Each plane has 2 channels. Probability of segmentation of disk and some relative position encoding parameter. The position encoding parameter helps the model combine the information from all the 3 models in the best way.

The 3D ensemble combines the best predictions form each single plane 2D model. Each model is better than the others at some specific regions of the disc and worse in others. A 2D model mask is better at the middle section (according to the direction of the normal of the plane) of the disc than in the endings (where the intersections are smaller). By putting more weight on the proper model (plane) prediction at each region, the 3D ensemble mask combines the best prediction from each of the models in each region. So the combined mask is better than any single plane 2D mask.

The other big effect of the 3D model is that it filters some prediction noise. 2D models sometimes predict false positives. There is a low probability that in a particular voxel more than 1 models have predicted false positives so the noise gets filtered. Single voxel or some small objects gets filtered too (Fig. 4).

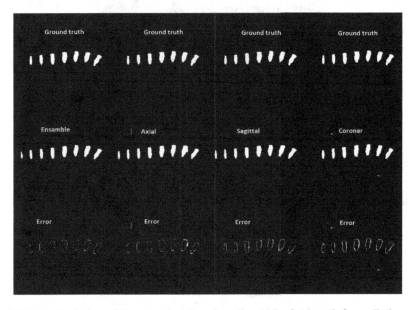

Fig. 4. The sagittal view of the ground truth and predicted binarized mask from all planes and combined with 3D ensemble.

Augmentation. In order to train a big model with a small dataset, extensive augmentations were used. Elastic whole image deformation – Take N × N uniform grid of points on the image, and chose a random direction vector for each point. Move each pixel in that direction with amplitude, proportional to f(inverse distance to the point). Tissue deformation – chose random points on the contour of the object and inside the object. Apply the elastic deformation on that points.

All the above augmentations, augment the image as well as the GT mask. Tissue brightness – change the values of the pixels lying in the ground-truth mask in some random direction. Noise – add white noise to each image, without changing the GT masks (Fig. 5).

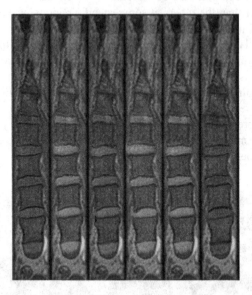

Fig. 5. The tissue deformation + brightness augmentation

3 Results

Challenge Result. Results achieved by 4-fold cross validation using the data provided by the organizers [7] are listed in Table 1.

Table 1. Comparison of single plane results vs 3D ensemble (cross validation).

2D planes used	Mean DICE
Sagittal	0.81
Axial	0.81
Coronal	0.77
Ensemble	0.915

As seen in Table 1, the 3D ensemble outputs 2 times less errors in the mask.

It is interesting that the middle discs have bigger dice than the first and the last. This phenomenon is observed in the other participants in the challenge too. May be the middle disc are "easier". We had big problems with detecting the 7-th disc (Th11–Th12) on some patients. Because only 7 discs were labeled in the GT, in some patients unlabeled discs appeared above the 7-th disc, which caused our classifier to get confused if it has to detect discs closer to the top end of the image or not. The problem was overcome by cropping the unlabeled discs out of the GT images during training. Test time is 3:10 s on a single GPU machine that can be reduced to 1:20 in batch mode. The model supports resolution of 512/512 that is 4 (2 × 2) times bigger than necessary for this particular set so test time can be further reduced (Table 2).

Table 2. Dice by disc (cross validation)

Metric	Disc_1	Disc_2	Disc_3	Disc_4	Disc_5	Disc_6	Disc_7	Mean
Dice	0.898695	0.925335	0.937724	0.929478	0.916675	0.907566	0.893001	0.915

During the cross validation we never observed detection of the sacrum. With this assumption we developed a simple filtration algorithm which takes the bottom 7 discs. But in test set evaluation the sacrum was detected in two of the patients which, led to missing the top disc completely and punishing the metrics of the bottom disc (Table 3).

Table 3. Dice by disc (challenge test set)

Metric	Disc_1	Disc_2	Disc_3	Disc_4	Disc_5	Disc_6	Disc_7	Mean
Dice	0.91568	0.916019	0.923087	0.917543	0.905131	0.897439	0.903565	0.9112

We calculated our expected test set dice metric without detecting the sacrum and missing the top disc (Table 4).

Table 4. Dice by disc without the 2 lost discs

Metric	Disc_1	Disc_2	Disc_3	Disc_4	Disc_5	Disc_6	Disc_7	Mean
Dice	0.91341	0.91602	0.92308	0.91754	0.90513	0.89744	0.90239	0.91072

Results in detecting disc herniation are as follows (Tables 5, 6 and 7).

Table 5. Herniated discs and slices performance

	Accuracy	Sensitivity	Specificity	Precision	TP	TN	FP	FN
Axial-Slice herniated	0.906	0.567	0.993	0.954	42	286	2	32
Disk herniated	0.890	0.750	0.975	0.947	18	39	1	6

Table 6. Localization of hernia top point

	Mean Abs error
Hernia X error on true positives	3 pix
Hernia Y error on true positives	2 pix
Hernia height error on all slices	1.3 pix

Table 7. Mask quality of different tissues (axial)

Tissue	IoU of mask for correctly detected objects
Disc	0.86
Disc and hernia	0.86
Dural sac	0.89
Hernia	0.66
Articular process	0.68
Ligament	0.62
Spinous process	0.73
Vertebrae	0.90
Whole disc	0.88

The performance of disc segmentation on our data is slightly worse than in the challenge because of the acquisition format that we use. The data in the challenge is 3D and has info for every voxel, while our data has slices spaced on bigger distance. The axial slices and sagittal slices are different sequences which are not strictly orthogonal to each other and to the coordinate system axes. 3D ensemble of the axial and sagittal slices is not straight forward. An experiment was undertaken to find the relation between the training set size and the validation set performance (Fig. 6).

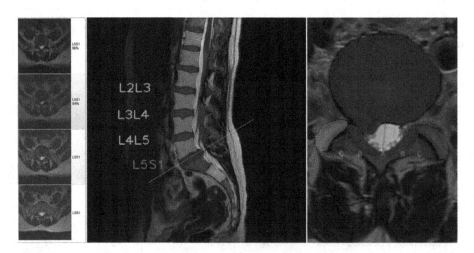

Fig. 6. Predicted masks of different tissues and probability of herniated disc. Automatic disk labeling.

4   Discussion

It seems like the ground truth masks of the 3D data are labeled only in the sagittal plane. The human annotator labeled each sagittal slice of the 3D matrix, producing 3D ground truth matrix concatenated from all the sagittal slices. This leads to strange artifacts when looking the 3D matrix form other perspectives.

The same thing is possible during prediction. We have 3 2D models each working on one of the three planes. Each model can make 1–2 pixel mistakes in the edge. So the 3D convolution, that combines the outputs of the three models, uses the prediction of each of the model in the region where it is most accurate. This way using the strengths of each of the model (Figs. 7 and 8).

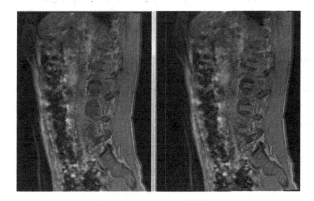

Fig. 7. Good looking ground truth disc segmentations in sagittal view.

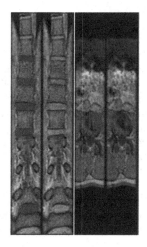

Fig. 8. Artifacts in ground truth masks viewed from plane which was not used during labeling.

The same thing is possible during prediction. We have 3 2D models each working on one of the three planes. Each model can make 1–2 pixel mistakes in the edge. So the 3D convolution, that combines the outputs of the three models, uses the prediction of each of the model in the region where it is most accurate. This way using the strengths of each of the models.

Problems with Detection. Although the mask quality of correctly detected objects is relatively good, there is a problem with detecting small objects. The most likely reason is the big feature map stride (8 × 8). When the stride is big, one feature map pixel corresponds to bigger area of original pixels. Instead of training one convolutional filter many times, one filter gets trained less times, but with more diverse set of positions of the smaller object in it. So there are a lot of places where the object did not appear in the filter's field of view. This leads to underfitting of the bigger convolutional filter and to underfitting of the detector.

5   Conclusion

Test accuracy was similar to the previously reported results using 3D convolutions on the test data of the previous challenge [8] although the algorithm was designed for 2D single-modality data. Training set accuracy is near 100% which can be expected as the complexity of the model is very big and definitely high variance is the current draw-back. Never the less we decided to not reduce the complexity as we believe bigger training set is necessary for reaching human level accuracy. So further test set accuracy improvements can be expected by increasing the training set. Our intention for the future development is to cover great variety of tissues and pathologies by acquiring an annotated training set of 500 patients. Part of them will be released to the scientific community.

References

1. Le Cun, Y., Bottou, L., Bengio, Y.: Reading checks with multilayer graph transformer networks. In: ICASSP 1997, vol. 1, pp. 151–154. IEEE (1997)
2. He, K., et al.: Deep residual learning for image recognition. In: CVPR 2016 (2016)
3. Hinton, G.E., et al.: Improving neural networks by preventing co-adaptation of feature detectors. Technical report. arXiv:1207.0580
4. Ioffe, S., Szegedy, C.: Batch normalization: accelerating deep network training by reducing internal covariate shift. CoRR abs/1502.03167 (2015)
5. Long, J., Shelhamer, E., Darrell, T.: Fully convolutional networks for semantic segmentation. arXiv:1411.4038 (2014)
6. Ronneberger, O., Fischer, P., Brox, T.: U-Net: convolutional networks for biomedical image segmentation. In: Navab, N., Hornegger, J., Wells, W.M., Frangi, A.F. (eds.) MICCAI 2015. LNCS, vol. 9351, pp. 234–241. Springer, Cham (2015). https://doi.org/10.1007/978-3-319-24574-4_28
7. Chen, C., Belavy, D., Zheng, G.: 3D intervertebral disc localization and segmentation from MR images by data-driven regression and classification. In: Wu, G., Zhang, D., Zhou, L. (eds.) MLMI 2014. LNCS, vol. 8679, pp. 50–58. Springer, Cham (2014). https://doi.org/10.1007/978-3-319-10581-9_7
8. Xiaomeng, L., et al.: 3D multi-scale FCN with random modality voxel dropout learning for intervertebral disc localization and segmentation from multi-modality MR images. Med. Image Anal. **45**, 41–54 (2018)

Evaluation and Comparison of Automatic Intervertebral Disc Localization and Segmentation methods with 3D Multi-modality MR Images: A Grand Challenge

Guodong Zeng[1(✉)], Daniel Belavy[2], Shuo Li[3], and Guoyan Zheng[1]

[1] Institute for Surgical Technology and Biomechanics, University of Bern, Bern, Switzerland
{guodong.zeng,guoyan.zheng}@istb.unibe.ch
[2] Deakin University, Geelong, Australia
[3] University of Western Ontario, London, Canada

Abstract. The localization and segmentation of Intervertebral Discs (IVDs) with 3D Multi-modality MR Images are critically important for spine disease diagnosis and measurements. Manual annotation is a tedious and laborious procedure. There exist automatic IVD localization and segmentation methods on multi-modality IVD MR images, but an objective comparison of such methods is lacking. Thus we organized the following challenge: Automatic Intervertebral Disc Localization and Segmentation from 3D Multi-modality MR Images, held at the 2018 International Conference on Medical Image Computing and Computer Assisted Intervention (MICCAI 2018). Our challenge ensures an objective comparison by running 8 submitted methods with docker container. Experimental results show that overall the best localization method achieves a mean localization distance of 0.77 mm and the best segmentation method achieves a mean Dice of 90.64% and a mean average absolute distance of 0.60 mm, respectively. This challenge still keeps open for future submission and provides an online platform for methods comparison.

Keywords: Intervertebral disc · MRI · Localization · Segmentation · Multi-modality · Challenge

1 Introduction

Degeneration of intervertebral discs (IVDs) has a strong association with low back pain (LBP) which is one of most prevalent health problems amongst population and a leading cause of disability [1]. Magnetic Resonance (MR) Imaging (MRI) is widely recognized as the imaging technique of choice for the assessment of lumbar IVD abnormalities due to its excellent soft tissue contrast and no ionizing radiation [2]. Thus, automated image analysis and quantification for

© Springer Nature Switzerland AG 2019
G. Zheng et al. (Eds.): CSI 2018, LNCS 11397, pp. 163–171, 2019.
https://doi.org/10.1007/978-3-030-13736-6_14

spinal diseases using MR images have drawn a lot of attention. Localization and segmentation are important steps before analysis and quantification. Previous works on disc degeneration were mainly done by manual segmentation, which is a time-consuming and tedious procedure. Automatic localization and segmentation of IVDs are highly preferred in clinical practice.

However, it is very difficult to directly compare different methods because they are usually evaluated on different datasets. Thus, objective evaluation and comparison are highly desired. For example, Zheng et al. [3] held a challenge on 3D IVD localization and segmentation in MICCAI 2015. But this challenge only investigated on single modality MR images, i.e., T2 MR data. Multi-modality MR images provide complementary information which can help improve recognition accuracy, and therefore have been utilized in many medical image analysis tasks. In this challenge, we investigate different methods working on four-modality IVD MR images acquired with Dixon protocol: fat, in-phase, opposed-phase and water modality MR image. The four multi-modality MR images of the same subject were acquired in the same space and thus are aligned with each other.

How to ensure objective and fair comparison is a big concern in organizing a challenge. In this challenge, all participants are required to submit a docker container of their method. A docker container includes codes and all dependencies so that others can re-run the method quickly and reliably on another computer. By doing this, all results of each participant were generated by running submitted containers on the challenge organizer's machine.

The paper is arranged as follows. We first present the challenge organization, rules for evaluation, image dataset and the established validation framework in Sect. 2. A summary of each submitted method will be described in Sect. 3. The validation results of each participant will be presented in Sect. 4, followed by conclusion in Sect. 5.

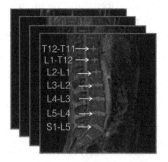
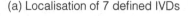
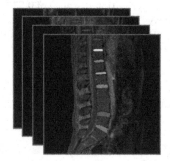

(a) Localisation of 7 defined IVDs   (b) Segmentation of 7 defined IVDs

Fig. 1. The 7 defined IVDs to be localized and segmented from each subject.

2   Challenge Setup

The aim of this challenge is to investigate fully automatic IVD localization and segmentation algorithms on a set of 3D Multi-modality MR images and to provide a standardized validation framework. The task for this challenge includes two parts: localization part and segmentation part. The task of localization part is to fully automatic localize the centers of 7 IVDs (T11-S1) for each test subject while the task of segmentation part is to fully automatic segment 7 disc regions T11-S1, which is illustrated in Fig. 1. For localization part, instead of detecting IVDs explicitly as a separate task, the centroids of each IVD generated from segmentation mask are recognized as the localization results.

2.1   Organization

Each participant could download the training data for method development after submitting a scanned copy of the signed registration form. For test data, both 3D MR images and corresponding ground truths will be only known to challenge organizers.

Participants should containerize their methods with Docker[1] and submit them to challenge organizers for evaluation. Containerized methods consist of codes and all dependencies so that challenge organizers can run all participants' methods quickly and reliably without complex development environment setup. By doing this, all prediction results were generated by running methods on challenge organiser's machine so that a fair comparison could be realized. More details about how to do the method containerization and to run the containers could be found at our challenge website[2], where an example in Python script was shown.

In the phase of testing, for each containerized method, it was run on each test subject one by one to get the segmentation result. To guarantee the running of containerized method is correct, challenge organizers sent the segmentation result of the first training subject back to the participants for verification. A desktop with a 3.6 GHz Intel(R) i7 CPU and a GTX 1080 Ti graphics card with 11 GB GPU memory was used to evaluate all submitted methods.

2.2   Description of Image Dataset

There are in total 24 sets of 3D multi-modality MRI data which contains at least 7 IVDs of the lower spine, collected from 12 subjects in two different stages in a study investigating the effect of prolonged bed rest (spaceflight simulation) on the lumbar intervertebral discs [4]. Each set of 3D multi-modality MRI data consists of four modality aligned high-resolution 3D MR images: in-phase, opposed-phase, fat and water images. Thus, in total we have 12 subjects × 2 stages × 4 modalities = 96 volume data.

---

[1]   https://www.docker.com.
[2]   https://ivdm3seg.weebly.com/methods.html.

All MR images were scanned with a 1.5-Tesla MRI scanner of Siemens (Siemens Health-care, Erlangen, Germany) using Dixon protocol [5]: slice thickness = 2.0 mm, pixel Spacing = 1.25 mm, repetition Time (TR) = 10.6 ms, echo time (TE) = 4.76 ms. The ground truth segmentation for each set of data were then manually annotated and were provided in the form of binary mask. All images (four volumes per patient) and binary masks (one binary volume per patient) are stored in the Neuroimaging Informatics Technology Initiative (NIFTI) file format.

During the challenge period, the organizer released training set of IVD challenge (8 subjects × 2 stages × 4modalities = 64 volume data). For test data, both MR images and ground truth segmentation will be only known to challenge organizer for independent evaluation and fair comparison (4 subjects × 2 stages × 4modalities = 64 volume data).

2.3   Rules for Evaluation

Submitted methods can generate multi-label segmentation or binary-label segmentation. We provide following rules for evaluation:

Multi-Label Prediction. If the prediction segmentation is not binary but with multiple labels, we will directly do the evaluation separately for seven IVDs in one test subject.

Binary-Label Prediction. If the prediction segmentation is binary, we first assign labels to each intervertebral disc based on ground truth segmentation and then do the evaluation. Specifically, the complete image space is spitted into 7 sections, corresponding to 7 intervertebral discs in the ground truth segmentation. Then we can do the evaluation similar as evaluation for multi-label prediction.

2.4   Evaluation Metrics

Three metrics were used to evaluate different methods: Mean Localization Distance (MLD) is used for localization task while Mean Dice Similarity Coefficients (MDSC) and Mean Average Surface Distance (MASD) are used for segmentation task. The details about how these three metrics are computed can be found as follows:

1. **Mean Localization Distance (MLD)**

For each IVD, we first calculate the localization distance (R) between the centroids of prediction and ground truth.

$$R = \sqrt{(\triangle x)^2 + (\triangle y)^2 + (\triangle z)^2} \qquad (1)$$

where $\triangle x$, $\triangle y$ and $\triangle z$ are the distances between the identified IVD centroids calculated from prediction and ground truth in x, y, z axis respectively.

After localization distance (R) was calculated, the MLD can be computed as follows:

$$MLD = \frac{\sum_{i=1}^{N_{images}} \sum_{j=1}^{N_{IVDs}} R_{ij}}{N_{images} N_{IVDs}} \quad (2)$$

where N_{images} is the number of test subjects, and N_{IVDs} is the number of IVDs in each test subject, i.e. 7 in our experiment. MLD indicates the measurement of average localization error for IVDs and lower value means better localization performance.

2. Mean Dice Similarity Coefficients (MDSC)

For each IVD, we first calculate Dice Similarity Coefficients (DSC) between prediction segmentation and ground truth segmentation, which is computed as follows:

$$DSC = \frac{2|A \cap B|}{|A| + |B|} \times 100\% \quad (3)$$

where A and B are foregrounds of prediction and ground truth segmentation respectively. And Mean Dice Similarity Coefficients (MDSC) is computed as below:

$$MDSC = \frac{\sum_{i=1}^{N_{images}} \sum_{j=1}^{N_{IVDs}} DSC_{ij}}{N_{images} N_{IVDs}} \quad (4)$$

where N_{images} is the number of test subjects, and N_{IVDs} is the number of IVDs in each test subject, i.e. 7 in our experiment. MDSC indicates the measurement of average overlap between the prediction and ground truth for IVDs and higher value means better segmentation performance.

3. Mean Average Surface Distance (MASD)

For each IVD, we first calculate Average Surface Distance (ASD) between prediction segmentation and ground truth segmentation. ASD calculation is implemented by medpy toolbox[3]. And Mean Average Surface Distance (MASD) is computed as below:

$$MASD = \frac{\sum_{i=1}^{N_{images}} \sum_{j=1}^{N_{IVDs}} ASD_{ij}}{N_{images} N_{IVDs}} \quad (5)$$

where N_{images} is the number of test subjects, and N_{IVDs} is the number of IVDs in each test subject, i.e. 7 in our experiment. MASD measures average surface distance between the prediction and ground truth for IVDs and lower value means better performance.

For each intervertebral disc, both the localization distance and ASD will be set as maximum value (458.24 mm) if the Dice value is less than 0.1% and additionally the number of segmented voxels assigned to this disc is smaller than 5% of the total voxels of the ground truth segmentation. In such a case, a method is regarded missing the segmentation of the disc completely.

---

[3] http://loli.github.io/medpy/.

2.5   Evaluation Ranking

The final ranking of all methods is based on three metrics described in Sect. 2.4. For each metric, we sort all methods (in total n methods) from best to worst. The best method will get a ranking score of 1, while the worst method get a ranking score of n. For each method, it will get an overall ranking score, which is the sum of its own ranking scores at each metrics. Lower overall ranking score indicates better performance. Finally, the final ranking of all methods will be in descending order by their overall ranking scores.

3   Methods

In total 8 teams submitted their methods and participated this challenge, but we only received 7 methods description. A brief summary of 7 methods is given below, in alphabetical order. Detailed method description and results of each team can be found at our challenge website[4].

1. changliu: a 2.5D U-Net-like [6] network which utilizes SEBottleneck [7] to achieve channel-wise attention and predicts segmentation mask of one slice from multiple-slice input (11 slices) [8].

2. gaoyunhecuhk: a 2D fully convolutional neural network which uses DenseNet [9] as the backbone network. Their network only down-samples for 2 times and uses Atrous Spatial Pyramid Pooling(ASPP) [10] to ensure a large receptive field [11].

3. livia: a UNet-like architecture which follows the multi-modality fusion strategy presented in [12], and all convolutional blocks are replaced by an Inception-like module and all convolutions are replaced by asymmetric convolutions [13].

4. lrde: the only method not using deep learning, but based on mathematical morphology operators which was driven by shape prior knowledge and their contrast in the different modalities [14].

5. mader: they first applied random forests with conditional random field (CRF) to detect 7 landmarks, i.e. the centroids of 7 IVDs. Then small fixed-size sections around each landmark were cropped and reoriented. At last, a V-Net [15] was trained to perform segmentation of IVDs [16].

6. smartsoft: Three 2D Unet-like neural networks were separately trained on 2d slice images in axial, sagittal, coronal axis respectively. The final segmentation result will be achieved by ensemble from three models [17].

7. ucsf_Claudia: V-Net was trained on full volumes to leverage the spatial context of the whole image [15]. The combination of weighted cross entropy (wce) loss and soft Dice loss was used. A 3D connected component analysis was employed to eliminate predicted volumes of less than 1200 voxels [18].

---

[4] https://ivdm3seg.weebly.com/miccai2018.html.

4   Experimental Results

The mean performance of each team is shown in Table 1. For each metric, there is an individual ranking and the final ranking is based on the sum of all metrics' ranking. The team changliu achieved best performance on all metrics, with a mean Dice Similarity Coefficients of 90.64%, a mean Average Surface Distance of 0.60 mm and a mean Localization Distance of 0.77 mm.

Table 1. Mean performance and ranking of each team on each metric. Metrics include MDSC, MASD and MLD. The final ranking is based on the sum of ranking on all metrics, in which lower value means better performance. Bold indicates the method performs best on that metric.

Final ranking (#)	TEAM	MDSC(%)	MASD (mm)	MLD (mm)	MDSC ranking value	MASD ranking value	MLD ranking value	Sum of ranking value
1	changliu	**90.64**	**0.60**	**0.77**	1	1	1	**3**
2	gaoyunhe_cuhk	90.58	0.61	0.78	2	2	2	6
3	ucsf_Claudia	89.71	0.74	0.86	3	4	3	10
4	livia	89.67	0.65	0.96	4	3	5	12
5	wanghuan	88.77	0.82	0.92	5	5	4	14
6	smartsoft	81.93	34.03	34.27	6	6	6	18
7	mader	66.42	108.19	108.41	7	7	7	21
8	lrde_01	24.35	319.53	319.81	8	8	8	24

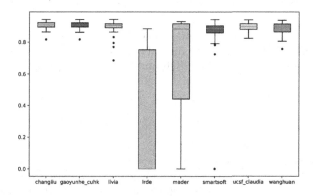

Fig. 2. Dice Similarity Coefficients (DSC) boxplot of 56 IVDs (8 test subjects × 7). The box shows the interquartile range (IQR) and extends from first quartile (Q1) to third quartile (Q3) values of the data, with a line at the median data. The whiskers extend up to 1.5 times of the IQR and those flier points beyond the whiskers are outliers.

And the following four teams, i.e. gaoyunhe_cuhk, ucsf_Claudia, livia and wanghuan also achieved good performance on both segmentation and localization tasks. Especially for the team gaoyunhe_cuhk, whose results show a very minor difference with the winner team changliu. Specifically, team gaoyunhe_cuhk reported a mean Dice Similarity Coefficients of 90.58%, a mean Average Surface Distance of 0.61 mm and a mean Localization Distance of 0.78 mm. But for the other three teams of smartsoft, mader, and lrde, they reported poor results on MDSC, MASD and MLD in this challenge.

Figure 2 shows boxplots of in total 56 IVDs (8 test subjects × 7) of each method on Dice Similarity Coefficients (DSC). As seen in Fig. 2, in terms of segmentation from team of mader and lrde, there are lots of completely failed cases whose DSC value are almost zero. Also, there are several such failed cases in the team of smartsoft. Figure 3 show boxplots of each method on Average Surface Distance (ASD) and Localization Distance (LD). Note that for each IVD, both the ASD and LD will be set as maximum value (458.24 mm) if a method is regarded missing the segmentation completely as mentioned in Sect. 2.4. As observed in Fig. 3, for teams of smartsoft, mader, and lrde, all of them reported some completely failed cases whose ASD and LD values are 458.24 mm.

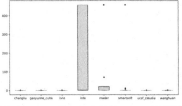
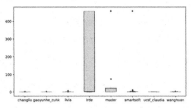

(a) Average Surface Distance (ASD) boxplot of IVDs

(b) Localization Distance (LD) boxplot of IVDs

Fig. 3. The boxes show the interquartile range (IQR) and extends from first quartile (Q1) to third quartile (Q3) values of the data, with a line at the median data. The whiskers extend up to 1.5 times of the IQR and those flier points beyond the whiskers are outliers.

5   Conclusion

This paper presents an objective comparison of state-of-the-art methods, which were submitted to the MICCAI 2018 challenge on Automatic Intervertebral Disc Localization and Segmentation from 3D Multi-modality MR Images. In total 8 teams submitted their results by docker container. The challenge organisers run their submitted methods on a local machine and then do the evaluation to ensure a fair comparison. The test data and ground truth are only known to the challenge organizers. The top-two ranking methods achieve similar results and the following three methods produce quite good results on both segmentation and localization tasks. The other 3 teams report poor results because their methods completely miss some IVDs. The organizers choose not to disclose the test data and corresponding ground truth, and the Challenge remains open for new submission in the future.

References

1. An, H.S., et al.: Introduction: disc degeneration: summary. Spine **29**(23), 2677–2678 (2004)
2. Emch, T.M., Modic, M.T.: Imaging of lumbar degenerative disk disease: history and current state. Skelet. Radiol. **40**(9), 1175 (2011)
3. Zheng, G., et al.: Evaluation and comparison of 3D intervertebral disc localization and segmentation methods for 3D T2 MR data: a grand challenge. Med. Image Anal. **35**, 327–344 (2017)
4. Belavỳ, D.L., Armbrecht, G., Felsenberg, D.: Incomplete recovery of lumbar intervertebral discs 2 years after 60-day bed rest. Spine **37**(14), 1245–1251 (2012)
5. Li, X., Dou, Q., Chen, H., Fu, C.-W., Heng, P.-A.: Multi-scale and modality dropout learning for intervertebral disc localization and segmentation. In: Yao, J., Vrtovec, T., Zheng, G., Frangi, A., Glocker, B., Li, S. (eds.) CSI 2016. LNCS, vol. 10182, pp. 85–91. Springer, Cham (2016). https://doi.org/10.1007/978-3-319-55050-3_8
6. Ronneberger, O., Fischer, P., Brox, T.: U-Net: convolutional networks for biomedical image segmentation. In: Navab, N., Hornegger, J., Wells, W.M., Frangi, A.F. (eds.) MICCAI 2015. LNCS, vol. 9351, pp. 234–241. Springer, Cham (2015). https://doi.org/10.1007/978-3-319-24574-4_28
7. Hu, J., Shen, L., Sun, G.: Squeeze-and-excitation networks. arXiv preprint arXiv:1709.01507 (2017)
8. Liu, C.: IVDM3Seg Challenge MICCAI 2018: Method Description of Team Changliu (2018). https://ivdm3seg.weebly.com/changliu.html
9. Huang, G., Liu, Z., Van Der Maaten, L., Weinberger, K.Q.: Densely connected convolutional networks. In: CVPR, vol. 1, p. 3 (2017)
10. Yang, M., Yu, K., Zhang, C., Li, Z., Yang, K.: DenseASPP for semantic segmentation in street scenes. In: Proceedings of the IEEE Conference on Computer Vision and Pattern Recognition, pp. 3684–3692 (2018)
11. Gao, Y.: IVDM3Seg Challenge MICCAI 2018: Method Description of Team gaoyunhe_cuhk (2018). https://ivdm3seg.weebly.com/gaoyunhe_cuhk.html
12. Dolz, J., Gopinath, K., Yuan, J., Lombaert, H., Desrosiers, C., Ayed, I.B.: HyperDense-net: a hyper-densely connected CNN for multi-modal image segmentation. arXiv preprint arXiv:1804.02967 (2018)
13. Dolz, J., Desrosiers, C., Ayed, I.B.: HD-UNet: hyper-dense UNet with asymmetric convolutions for multi-modal intervertebral disc segmentation (2018). https://ivdm3seg.weebly.com/livia.html
14. Carlinet, E., Géraud, T.: Intervertebral Disc Segmentation Using Mathematical Morphology (2018). https://ivdm3seg.weebly.com/lrde.html
15. Milletari, F., Navab, N., Ahmadi, S.A.: V-net: fully convolutional neural networks for volumetric medical image segmentation. In: 2016 Fourth International Conference on 3D Vision (3DV), pp. 565–571. IEEE (2016)
16. Mader, A.O., Lorenz, C., Meyer, C.: Segmenting Labeled Intervertebral Discs in Multi Modality MR Images (2018). https://ivdm3seg.weebly.com/mader.html
17. Georgiev, N., Asenov, A.: Automatic Segmentation of Lumbar Spine 3D MRI Using Ensemble of 2D Algorithms (2018). https://ivdm3seg.weebly.com/smartsoft.html
18. Iriondo, C., Girard, M.: Vesalius: VNet-based fully automatic segmentation of intervertebral discs in multimodality MR images (2018). https://ivdm3seg.weebly.com/ucsf_claudia.html

Short Papers

Vesalius: VNet-Based Fully Automatic Segmentation of Intervertebral Discs in Multimodality MR Images

Claudia Iriondo[1,2(✉)] and Michael Girard[2,3]

[1] Department of Bioengineering, University of California, Berkeley,
Berkeley, CA, USA
iriondo@berkeley.edu
[2] Department of Radiology and Biomedical Imaging, University of California,
San Francisco, San Francisco, CA, USA
michael.girard@ucsf.edu
[3] Center for Digital Health Innovation, University of California, San Francisco,
San Francisco, CA, USA

Abstract. Named after Andreas Vesalius (1914–1964) for his landmark description of the intervertebral discs, Vesalius is a VNet-based method for fully automatic segmentation of intervertebral discs T11/T12 to L5/S1 in sagittal Dixon MR sequences. Our method uses aggressive data augmentation, transfer learning from a T2 weighted MR dataset, a fully convolutional VNet architecture trained on full resolution image volumes, and model ensembling to smoothly segment intervertebral discs with up to 0.9285 Dice in our preliminary tests.

Keywords: Spine · Intervertebral disc · Segmentation · VNet

1 Data Splitting

As mentioned in the IVDM3seg challenge description, data released for method development consisted of 8 patients scanned at two timepoints. Leakage between training and testing data should be avoided; the network should be discouraged from "memorizing" specific patients' intervertebral discs during training. Volumes were paired based on structural similarity and restricted to the same training/testing group. Augmentations of these volumes were also contained to the same group. Train test split was 14/2 and leave-one-out-cross validation was performed by shuffling training and testing groups while respecting patient divisions, creating a total of 8 unique data folds.

2 Data Augmentation and Preprocessing

The full dataset was augmented 38X using a combination of 3D rotation, 3D affine transforms, and 3D elastic deformations and stored offline. These deformations were designed to mimic variable patient positioning, spinal curvature, disc size, and disc shape.

© Springer Nature Switzerland AG 2019
G. Zheng et al. (Eds.): CSI 2018, LNCS 11397, pp. 175–177, 2019.
https://doi.org/10.1007/978-3-030-13736-6

Volumes and segmentation masks were resampled to isotropic dimensions, augmented, then resampled back to their original dimensions. Volumes and masks were interpolated using cubic interpolation and masks defined by a 0.5 threshold. Intensities were normalized to zero mean, unit variance on a per volume, per channel basis.

3   Network Structure and Training Details

A 3D VNet architecture was implemented in Tensorflow using Python (algorithm [1], graph [2]) and trained end-to-end. VNet is a fully convolutional neural network architecture consisting of sequential 3D strided convolutional downsampling units and a transpose convolution upsampling path with skip connections concatenated at each resolution. By training the network with our full volumes, instead of patches, we were able to leverage the spatial context of the whole image to predict our binary segmentation mask. Our final network took a 4 channel input, one channel per modality, expanded to 16 channels at the first layer, and doubled in channels every subsequent level for a total of 256 channels at the bottom of the network. The networks 4 levels had 1,2,3,3 convolutions respectively and 3 convolutions at the bottom level with ReLu activations.

Our loss metric combined weighted cross entropy (wce) loss and soft Dice loss. Although the contribution of weighted cross entropy in the combined loss function was relatively small (wce scaled by 0.017 and added to soft Dice), our combined loss metric was successful in addressing the imbalance of foreground to background voxels.

Finally, each network was trained for 25 epochs (approximately 8 h, although convergence was seen within 30 min) on a single Nvidia Titan X GPU using gradient descent optimizer with exponential learning rate decay.

4   Transfer Learning

Networks underwent supervised pre-training for 25 epochs on a single-channel T2 weighted dataset from a previous MICCAI competition [3]. The T2w dataset was cropped to match the field of view and resolution of the Dixon sequence, augmented using the techniques described above, and broadcast to four input channels to match the dimensions. Learned weights were used for weight initialization of our VNet.

5   Hyperparameter Tuning and Ensembling

A random search of 60 unique combinations of hyperparameters was performed. Due to computational restrictions, the search was only performed on 1 of the 8 data folds. The hyperparameter set with the highest and most stable test Dice accuracy and visually smoothest segmentation was selected. Finally, 8 models were trained, each on a unique data fold, using this hyperparameter set (initial learning rate = 0.029, decay steps/decay rate = 3500/0.0700, background voxel weight wce = 0.014, foreground voxel weight wce = 1.0, wce contribution to loss = 0.017, batch size = 1, dropout = 0.80).

The input image is loaded, each channel normalized to zero mean unit variance, and it is run through inference of models 1 through 8. The logits of all models are averaged and used for prediction. In the case of a "missing" prediction for T11/T12 disc, the input is flipped across axis = 0 and run through the inference again, and auxiliary predictions are used for segmentation.

6   Post-processing

A 3D connected component analysis was used to eliminate predicted volumes of less than 1200 voxels. Based on our observation of the manual segmentation ground truth, segmentations appeared to be processed slice-wise in the sagittal plane. Partial volume effect is a known problem in determining boundaries for segmentation of "bookend" slices. To address this issue, a 2D connected component analysis was performed on the bookend sagittal slices to remove any segmentations smaller than 25 pixels (size of smallest manually drawn ROI). Finally, 3D connected components were labeled bottom up with background assigned a value of 0, disc L5/S1 assigned a value of 1, L4/L5 2 and so on. The center of the disk is defined as the centroid of each 3D connected component.

References

1. Milletari, F., Navab, N., Ahmadi, S.: V-Net: Fully Convolutional Neural Networks for Volumetric Medical Image Segmentation (2016). https://arxiv.org/abs/1606.04797
2. Monteiro, M.: https://github.com/MiguelMonteiro/VNet-Tensorflow. Accessed May 2018
3. Zheng, G., et al.: Evaluation and comparison of 3D intervertebral disc localization and segmentation methods for 3D T2 MR data: a grand challenge. Med Image Anal. (2017)

Segmenting Labeled Intervertebral Discs in Multi Modality MR Images

Alexander Oliver Mader[1,2,3(✉)], Cristian Lorenz[3], and Carsten Meyer[1,2,3]

[1] Institute of Computer Science,
Kiel University of Applied Sciences, Kiel, Germany
[2] Department of Computer Science, Faculty of Engineering,
Kiel University, Kiel, Germany
[3] Department of Digital Imaging,
Philips Research Hamburg, Hamburg, Germany
alexander.o.mader@fh-kiel.de

1 Method

The task it so segment seven well-defined intervertebral discs (IVDs) in multi modality MR images. For this we propose a method specifically designed to be trained on a very small training set. The key idea is to reorient sections around the individual IVDs to a standard orientation in order to be efficiently segmented by an IVD-agnostic V-Net [2]. This leads to the following four step approach, as illustrated in Fig. 1.

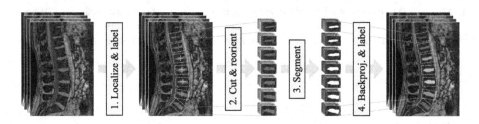

Fig. 1. Illustration of our four step approach to predict labeled IVD segmentations.

1.1 Localizing and Labeling IVDs

First, we use our approach proposed in [1] to localize and label the IVD's center of mass positions. It is a general method to localize and label arbitrary key points by applying landmark-specific localizers (e.g., random forests or FCNs, here random forests) followed by a conditional random field (CRF) to model the global shape. It has been applied to different dimensionalities (2D, 3D) and modalities (X-ray, CT) already, but has neither been applied so far to MR images nor to a multi modality setup. Here, we extend our method to work with multi modality (i.e., multi-channel) MR images by correspondingly increasing the depth of

© Springer Nature Switzerland AG 2019
G. Zheng et al. (Eds.): CSI 2018, LNCS 11397, pp. 178–180, 2019.
https://doi.org/10.1007/978-3-030-13736-6

the image volume (4 in this case instead of a single channel volume). An additional modification compared to our previous work applies to the CRF: Instead of using the proposed binary potentials, we use ternary potentials to increase the rotation and scaling invariance in combination with unary potentials related to the localizers. I.e., we use a Gaussian distribution to model the ratio between two distances and a von Mises distribution to model the relative angle between two vectors projected to one plane. Applying this method we obtain a labeled localization hypothesis for each IVD.

1.2 Sampling Reoriented IVD Sections

Given the IVD locations predicted by the previous step, we sample small reoriented fixed-size sections around each prediction. The size ($6 \times 5 \times 3$ cm) is chosen such that the classes are balanced and the sections are reoriented such that the IVDs are level inside the sections (see second step in Fig. 1). PCA was applied to the training segmentations to find the standard orientation of each IVD.

1.3 Segmenting IVDs

As third step, we perform the actual segmentation of the disc tissue using the fully convolutional network V-Net [2]. We use the standard architecture and train it using the setup proposed by the authors. A mini-batch size of 7 is used and the optimization is carried out for 5000 epochs. To tackle the problem of few training cases, we train one label agnostic model to segment all seven IVD sections, effectively using the network to discriminate disc tissue from non-disc tissue (2-class problem instead of 8-class problem). To further accelerate the performance, we increase the training set size even more by a factor of 10 using data augmentation in the form of translation and rotation. Note that histogram matching is performed prior segmentation as data normalization.

Finally, the resulting segmentations are back-projected into the original label space and relabeled according to the label predicted by the CRF in first step.

1.4 Evaluation

We used an 8-fold cross validation setup (14 training images, 2 test images) to estimate essential parameters and to evaluate the training performance. On average, our method achieves a Dice coefficient of 0.894 and a mean surface distance of 0.45 mm, while processing one image in (on average) less than 10 s. For testing, we use an ensemble of our 8 models to improve robustness.

Acknowledgements. This work has been financially supported by the Federal Ministry of Education and Research under the grant 03FH013IX5. The liability for the content of this work lies with the authors.

References

1. Mader, A.O., et al.: Detection and localization of landmarks in the lower extremities using an automatically learned conditional random field. In: Cardoso, M.J., et al. (eds.) GRAIL/MFCA/MICGen -2017. LNCS, vol. 10551, pp. 64–75. Springer, Cham (2017). https://doi.org/10.1007/978-3-319-67675-3_7
2. Milletari, F., Navab, N., Ahmadi, S.A.: V-net: fully convolutional neural networks for volumetric medical image segmentation. In: 3DV, pp. 565–571. IEEE (2016)

Author Index

Printed in the United States
By Bookmasters